Urban Livelihoods and Food and Nutrition Security in Greater Accra, Ghana

Daniel Maxwell

Carol Levin

Margaret Armar-Klemesu

Marie Ruel

Saul Morris

Clement Ahiadeke

IFPRI NMIMR World Health Organization

International Food Policy Research Institute
Noguchi Memorial Institute for Medical Research
World Health Organization

Library of Congress Cataloging-in-Publication Data

Urban livelihoods and food and nutrition security in Greater Accra, Ghana / Daniel Maxwell . . . [et al.].
p. cm. — (Rearch report ; 112)
"The International Food Policy Research Institute; In collaboration with the Noguchi Memorial Institute for Medical Research and The World Health Organization."
"April 2000."
Includes bibliographical references.
ISBN 0-89629-115-4
1. Nutrition surveys—Ghana. I. Maxwell, Daniel. II. Research report (International Food Policy Research Institute); 112.

TX360.G4 U73 2000
363.8'09667—dc21 99-087101

Contents

Tables

Figures

Foreword

The population of the developing world is becoming more urban, with the urban population projected to double from 1.7 billion in 1995 to 3.4 billion in 2020. Although malnutrition and poverty are still more prevalent in rural areas today, rising deprivation in urban areas now presents a serious challenge in developing countries—not simply a concern for the future.

In 1996, IFPRI started a program of research on urban challenges to food and nutrition security to better understand trends in urban poverty, food insecurity, and malnutrition and their determinants and interrelationships. A component of this work, which uses available literature and empirical data on poverty and children's nutritional status shows that in fact the locus of poverty and malnutrition is shifting from rural to urban areas. The absolute number of poor as well as the urban share of the poor and malnourished is increasing in many countries. To better understand the issues, IFPRI implemented several research projects to explore the interactions between urban livelihoods, poverty, food security, and health and nutrition outcomes.

The results, the first to emerge from this research program, provide important insights into the challenges that urban households face. Based on the evidence presented here, policymakers and urban planners should act now to address problems of urban food insecurity and malnutrition. The authors present a number of policy and program recommendations that have wide applications for the many countries facing rapid urban population growth and the accompanying problems of food insecurity and malnutrition among the poor.

Per Pinstrup-Andersen
Director General

Acknowledgments

This study is a collaborative effort of the Noguchi Memorial Institute for Medical Research (NMIMR) of the University if Ghana, the International Food Policy Research Institute (IFPRI), and the World Health Organization (WHO), in collaboration with Ghanaian nongovernmental organizations (NGOs) on various aspects of the study. A companion report will be published by WHO in early 2000 (*WHO Multi-Country Study on Improving Household Food and Nutrition Security for the Vulnerable: Ghana. Achieving Urban Food and Nutrition Security for the Vulnerable in Greater Accra.* Geneva: WHO, 2000. WHO/NHD/00.2).

Additional financial support was provided by several organizations, including the Rockefeller Foundation, the International Development Research Centre (IDRC), and the Canadian International Development Agency (CIDA). We thank Chizuru Nishida of WHO, Luc Mougeot of IDRC, and Anne Lavender and Richard Beattie of CIDA for their interest in and support of the study.

Many institutions collaborated on some elements of the study. These include the Accra Metropolitan Assembly (AMA), the Tema Municipal Assembly, the Ga District Assembly, the National Development Planning Commission, the Institute for Statistical Social and Economic Research (University of Ghana), the Lands Commission, the Accra Sustainable Programme, the Environmental Protection Agency, the Ministry of Food and Agriculture, CENCOSAD, May Day Rural Project, the La Farmer's Association, the Greater Accra Vegetable Grower's Association, and CARE International. We thank each of these collaborating institutions for their contributions to the study.

There are too many individuals in this list of institutions to name them all, but special thanks go to Nat Nunoo-Amarteifio, chief executive of the AMA; James Annorbah Sarpei of CENCOSAD; Ken Williams of the United Nations Children's Fund (UNICEF); Rosanna Agble of the Ministry of Health; Rosetta Tetebo of the Ministry of Food and Agriculture; Dr. Twum-Baah and Mr. Bannerman of the Ghana Statistical Service; Odame Larbi of the Lands Commission; Ben Doe and Doris Tetteh of the Accra Sustainable Programme; Samual Anku of the Environmental Protection Agency; S. N. A. Attoh, the Ga District agricultural officer; E. O. Laryea of May Day Project; and many other public and NGO officials.

At Noguchi Memorial Institute for Medical Research, we specifically thank the director, Francis Nkrumah, for his unflagging support of the study, as well as Lucy Brakohiapa, Anna Mills, Gloria Folson, and members of the staff of the nutrition unit, and Patience Akpedonu of the bacteriology unit.

At the International Food Policy Research Institute, we thank the director of the Food Consumption and Nutrition Division, Lawrence Haddad, for all his contributions of time, effort (and core funds) to the study, as well as Lynette Aspillera, James Garrett, Jay Willis, Haydee Lemus, and other staff members of the Food Cosumption and Nutrition Division. We thank John Hoddinott of IFPRI, Jane Pryer of the London School of Hygiene and Tropical Medicine, and Stacy Gage of USAID for reviewing the manuscript.

The field staff of the project are too many to name individually, but we especially thank the long-term research support staff, including Charlotte Mensah, Sawudatu Zakariah, Grace Mary Lamptey, and Godfred Egbi. Mercy Krow, Frederick Vuvor, and John Yeyie were field supervisors for the survey. Emmanuel Amokwandoh led the data entry team. The entire survey field team consisted of some 35 people, including the supervisors just named, enumerators, anthropometry teams, and drivers. We are grateful to each of them.

Each of us thanks our families for their understanding and support, and for putting up with occasional excessive absence from familial duties, due to the long hours devoted to the study. And last but not least, we thank the thousands of individual Accra residents who spared us the time answer our seemingly endless questions. We hope the study will be of benefit to them.

Summary

The dramatic growth of cities in the developing world has brought with it a new challenge—widespread and increasing urban poverty. However, efforts to address the unique problems of urban poverty lag far behind the growth of the problems themselves. Antipoverty initiatives have traditionally targeted rural areas, which were presumed to have been worse off than urban areas. But the problems of poor city dwellers have become more pressing, including the issues of how the urban poor earn their livelihoods and the ways in which this affects key indicators of human welfare, such as food security and nutrition, especially of children.

This report examines the nature of urban poverty and how it relates to food insecurity and malnutrition in Accra, Ghana. By exploring the major determinants of food security and nutritional status, it develops indicators that are appropriate in an urban context, identifies vulnerable groups within the city, and suggests policies and programs to improve the lives of the urban poor.

The Accra Urban Food and Nutrition Study was a collaborative effort of the International Food Policy Research Institute, the Noguchi Memorial Institute of Medical Research, located in Accra, and the World Health Organization. The 1996–97 study included participatory community studies, household case studies, a household survey, and follow-up interviews and focus groups. The analysis of the information gleaned from these activities is based on a blend of two conceptual frameworks—one for livelihood security and one for child nutritional status. Children's nutritional status is determined by their food intake, health, and the care they receive. This report seeks to determine how the strategies employed by the urban poor to secure their livelihoods affect the household's food security; the care of household members, especially children; and the resulting health and nutrition outcomes. Household food consumption data collected include the "street foods" purchased from vendors. The hygiene behaviors practiced, the local sanitation conditions, and behaviors related to feeding and caring for children are all studied to determine their contributions to the high rates of malnutrition.

Urban livelihoods are complex and not easily characterized. Urban households rely heavily on their labor for income. Men's and women's activities are very different, however. Men are likely to be involved in skilled or unskilled labor—sometimes self-employed, sometimes as wage laborers—and some have clerical or professional jobs. Women are more likely to engage in petty trade or street food vending, where they earn far less than men. Because households headed by males have more resources for earning income and fewer dependents, they tend to have higher per capita incomes than female-headed households.

Both individuals and households strive to diversify their income sources. For the survey sample as a whole, the mean number of income-generating activities per household was found to be only 1.9, and it was significantly lower for female-headed households. The research team observed much more income diversification than the survey results indicate, but many of these income resources were short term in nature.

Urban agriculture does not play as large a role in household livelihood strategies within the city of Accra as in some other African cities, but it is of critical importance in the peri-urban areas around the city. Agriculture as a source of livelihood is increasingly vulnerable as the city physically expands, destroying farmland.

The people of Accra are heavily reliant on the urban market for access to food. More than 90 percent of all food consumed is purchased for cash, about 6 percent comes from gifts, 1 percent is given to a worker in lieu of wages, and 1 percent is home-produced. Even among households engaged in urban agriculture, only about 7 percent of food (in value terms) is home-produced. Overall, 32 percent of the food budget is spent on prepared foods, but the poor spend nearly 40 percent of their food budget on street foods. A correspondingly high proportion of calories—roughly 30 percent for the entire sample—comes from street foods.

Interhousehold transfers of money play a crucial role in livelihood strategies, especially for low-income households, indigenous communities, and for female-headed households. Most of this transfer income is spent on personal and household consumption needs.

Urban households spend more than half of their budgets on food, but nearly one-fifth of the households spend more than 70 percent of their income on food. Housing takes up a surprisingly small share of the total household budget because many of the people surveyed live in family compounds that they neither own nor rent.

Based on the calories available to household members per day (2,640 kilocalories per adult equivalent unit), about 40 percent of households in the sample are food-insecure. When the measure of food insecurity takes into consideration both the number of calories available and the share of the total household budget devoted to food, 24 percent are classified as food insecure and 40 percent as vulnerable; these are mostly among the lowest income groups. People who live in female-headed households consume more calories, but larger shares of the household budgets go to acquire food. Therefore, female-headed households and individuals in occupations that are predominantly female, such as petty trading and food vending, are the most vulnerable to food price rises or income shocks.

From 1988 to 1993 the nutritional status of children generally improved, but from 1993 to 1997 it again deteriorated. Among children 3 to 36 months old, the prevalence of stunting (low height-for-age) was 17.6 percent in the latter period. The prevalence of wasting (low weight-for-height) was 5.3 percent.

Life in urban areas presents special challenges for the provision of adequate care. The trade-offs women face between their productive and reproductive roles are likely to be more acute in urban than in rural areas. In Accra, about two-thirds of all primary caregivers of young children (usually their mothers) engage in some kind of income-generating activity. Most caregivers work away from home and work very long hours. Nevertheless, among those who work, more than half still look after their children full time, taking them to the marketplace or wherever they work. Mothers of young children perceive that their ability to care for their children may be adversely affected while working, but they also know that they must earn an income to provide for their children. Results here suggest that many working women are able to cope, avoiding adverse effects on their children.

According to the survey, child feeding practices are less than ideal in Accra. Although breast feeding is the norm, use of prelacteal feeds and complementary foods and liquids during the first four months is widespread. Use of health services for immunization and growth monitoring, however, is high, probably a reflection of the availability and promotion of these services in the city. As expected, children from households with higher incomes have access to more and better quality food and have better health.

Care practices and behaviors are not significantly improved in higher-income households, however. Maternal schooling is the determinant most strongly associated with good care. This study finds that mother's education clearly matters. More education for women is associated with higher levels of household food availability, higher quality diets, better care practices and behaviors, and better nutritional outcomes.

Despite clear differences in the appearance and composition of urban neighborhoods, the variations in income and human welfare between the areas surveyed are less significant than those within an area. For programs aimed at reducing urban poverty and increasing food and nutrition security, this implies that simple geographic targeting is not sufficient. Virtually all the variation is at the household level, not the community level. To effectively intervene, at-risk households and individuals will have to be identified through means other than their neighborhood; targeting strategies will be needed to identify vulnerable groups wherever they are located.

The findings of this study have important policy implications for reducing urban poverty and vulnerability. But to do so several preconditions must be met. Governments must accept that rapid urban growth is a reality in Sub-Saharan Africa. Although poverty is predominantly a rural problem in Ghana, urban poverty must be recognized. National policies must address the needs of different categories of vulnerable groups, such as female-headed households. Education of girls is a good investment for reducing poverty in the future. For other livelihood groups, vulnerability stems from poor employment opportunities, lack of access to credit, and the regulatory environment, which inhibits the activities of the urban self-employed.

The rapid proliferation of traders and vendors of street foods will require new approaches by municipal authorities, emphasizing participation and collaboration rather than control. Strengthening trader or street food vendor associations would help to develop self-regulatory mechanisms and give a political voice to small-scale entrepreneurs.

CHAPTER 1

Urban Poverty: A New Priority

Poverty, food insecurity, and malnutrition in Africa were for decades viewed as largely—if not entirely—rural problems. At the end of the twentieth century, however, rapid urbanization in Sub-Saharan Africa has resulted in urban poverty severe enough to jeopardize livelihoods and food and nutrition security. The urban population, a tiny fraction of the region's residents in 1950, is now approaching 40 percent of the total and is expected to exceed 50 percent early in the twenty-first century (UNCHS 1996). This urban growth has brought with it a host of problems, including unemployment and underemployment, a burgeoning informal sector, deteriorating infrastructure and service delivery capacity, overcrowding and environmental degradation, and an acute housing shortage (Stren, White, and Whitney 1992; Mabogunje 1994; Becker, Jamer, and Morrison 1994; UNCHS 1996).

These issues have been broadly reviewed in the 1990s (Ruel et al. 1998; von Braun et al. 1993; Atkinson 1992). Only a few empirical studies have undertaken a comprehensive analysis in an urban context, however (Tabatabai 1993; Gebre 1993). Recent research has made urban poverty a priority on the political agenda of donors and national government (Amis 1995; OECD 1995; Moser 1996; Stren, White, and Whitney 1992; de Haan 1997; Ruel et al. 1998). Recent analyses have shown, for instance, that urban poverty is not only growing rapidly but has tended to be underestimated in the past (Haddad, Ruel, and Garrett 1999; Satterthwaite 1995).

Specific policy attention to issues of urban poverty such as food security and nutrition has lagged behind the research, despite the demonstrated need. Earlier research showed that 60–80 percent of the total household budget of the urban poor is spent on food (Tabatabai 1993; Gebre 1993). This finding makes it likely that urban poverty will be manifested at least in part as a food insecurity problem. Within the West African region, urban food security—and the dearth of research on the topic—has been recognized as a growing problem (Onibokun 1994).

Urban poverty is unique. The valuable policy and programmatic lessons generated by decades of work in rural Africa may not be directly applicable to cities, for several reasons. First, urban life has a different effect on all the major determinants of nutritional status than rural life does, including livelihoods, food access, dietary intake, the capacity of households to provide adequate care for all members,[1] and environmental conditions (such as crowding) that influence health and the incidence of illness (Ruel et al. 1998). Second, vulnerable groups in cities often have fewer informal safety nets (kinship and community networks), and formal safety nets for urban populations have largely collapsed or been dismantled (de Haan 1997; Moser 1996). Third, the macroeconomic policies of many African states in the late 1980s and 1990s are widely believed to have had a deleterious effect on wage-dependent urban workers. These policies have created a new class of vulnerable people, and much of this class is in urban areas—a finding echoed by other recent research on the impact of structural adjustment in Sub-Saharan Africa (Demery and Squire 1996; Sahn, Dorosh, and Younger 1996; Mabogunje 1994; Becker, Jamer, and Morrison 1994).

Urban development and the role of cities on national development have long been controversial topics in development theory. Modernization theory equated urbanization with industrialization and treated both as desirable goals of development (Todaro 1977). Populist revision of modernization theory and neo-Marxist theory in the 1970s and 1980s reversed this view, noting that urbanization in Africa was not necessarily associated with industrialization, but was an extractive—even "parasitic"—process that undermined agriculture and rural development (Baker and Pedersen 1992). A famous and enduring treatise by Lipton (1977) proposed rural-urban differences as a central analytical category in the study of poverty and introduced the concept of "urban bias," or the notion that urban populations are structurally privileged over their rural counterparts.

Urban bias became one of the intellectual cornerstones of economic reforms in Africa in the 1980s (Bates 1981; World Bank 1981). There is little doubt that many of the mechanisms Bates analyzed—markets, imports and exports, exchange rates, formal employment, and services—did give an economic and political advantage to certain social groups, most of them urban. The urban bias debate tended to obscure the analysis of urban poverty, and even the recognition that such poverty existed, for some time.

New analyses are challenging the notion of urban bias, however. A recent report by the Organisation for Economic Co-operation and Development (OECD) (1995) describes the effects of shocks on growing urban populations. The report notes that West Africa is suffering from two major shocks: rapid population growth and "brutal" exposure to world markets. The population of West Africa will roughly double between 1995 and 2020, and about two-thirds of this growth is projected to take place in cities. "Massive" growth in the urban informal sector can be expected over the next 25 years. Social inequalities are likely to increase over the same period in both urban and rural areas, but nowhere more than in the big cities.

West Africa's experience is not unique. The impact of structural adjustment is being felt throughout the African continent—in particular by urban populations

[1] Care is the provision in the household and the community of time, attention, and support to meet the physical, mental, and social needs of the growing child and other household members (ICN 1993).

(OECD 1995). According to the OECD, the effects of structural adjustment on urban areas include

- *higher food prices,* the result of liberalized agricultural output markets and the lifting of subsidies and state control over grains and other food products;
- *higher prices for imported goods* caused by the liberalization of imports and exports;
- *growing joblessness among middle-class residents,* many of whom have been pushed out by the privatization and downsizing of the civil service;
- *lower wages,* the result of increasingly competitive labor markets; and
- *reductions in basic health, education, and other social services* as governments reduce expenditures.

Most of these reforms have been necessary. They are designed to stimulate agricultural productivity, lay the foundation for renewed growth, and, ironically, reduce urban bias. But structural adjustment has also created a new class of vulnerable people, many of them in urban areas. Other recent research on the impacts of structural adjustment in Sub-Saharan Africa echo these findings (Demery and Squire 1996; Sahn, Dorosh, and Younger 1996). Research also suggests that while structural adjustment policies have improved agricultural incentives, they have not significantly altered the pattern of rural-urban migration (OECD 1995; Becker, Jamer, and Morrison 1994).

Greater Accra, Ghana: A Case Study in Urban Poverty

Accra offers a compelling case study of the contemporary impact of urban life on the livelihoods, food security, and nutritional status of its people. The Accra Urban Food and Nutrition Study was a collaborative effort between IFPRI, the Noguchi Institute of Medical Research, and the World Health Organization to assess the nature of urban poverty and the relationship between urban poverty and food insecurity or malnutrition in Accra, Ghana, in 1996–97. By exploring the major determinants of food security and nutrition status, the study develops indicators of food and livelihood security that are appropriate for an urban setting. The study consists of participatory community studies, household case studies, a household survey carried out in 19 areas of Greater Accra Metropolitan Area, and follow-up interviews and focus groups.

The Economic Context

Ghana's economy underwent a long period of decline from 1965 to 1983. In many ways this decline was a classic example of the failure of development policy, complete with falling production, decaying infrastructure, overvalued exchange rates (and therefore implicit taxes on exports), and declining investment and high inflation. Food prices increased steadily and standards of living declined. In several instances, urban dwellers experienced severe food shortages (Kraus 1988; Commander, Howell, and Seini 1989). Political protests against food shortages and price hikes were linked to at least two coups, although many protests were directed at food traders rather than the government. This situation came to a head in 1982–83, when a severe nationwide drought drastically reduced harvests and triggered massive food shortages. The country avoided widespread famine, but Ghanaians' nutritional status declined severely nationwide (Tabatabai 1988).

The Economic Recovery Programme, Ghana's structural adjustment program, began in 1983. The program has been widely perceived as successful (Alderman 1994), although inflation has been high since 1992, undermining much of the recovery effort (ISSER 1997). Agricultural production increased quickly, despite variances in annual production (which have persisted since 1984) and steep seasonal price fluctuations. Overall GDP growth in the 1990s has ranged between 4 and 5 percent (ISSER 1997). But many groups have yet to benefit significantly from the recovery, and few have been able to recover their precrisis standard of living.

Population

In 1997 the population of greater Accra was estimated to be roughly 2.3–2.4 million people. The projected overall population growth rate in the study area at the time of the study was roughly 4.7 percent per year (Table 1). Accra itself covers 17,362.4 hectares, so that its mean population density at the time of the survey was 100 people per hectare. Actual population densities vary from as few as 20 people per hectare in the new high-income areas to as many as 500 people per hectare in the most densely populated low-income neighborhoods (Ghana-MLG 1992).

Table 1—Population and growth rates for greater Accra

Location	1960	1970	1984	1995[a]	2000[a]
			(thousands)		
Population					
Accra	388	637	969	1,513	1,843
Tema	27	102	191	350	459
Ga District	34	66	133	262	348
Total	449	805	1,293	2,216	2,650
			(percent)		
Growth rate					
Accra	...	5.1	3.1	4.0	4.1
Tema	...	14.2	4.5	5.8	5.9
Ga District	...	6.9	5.3	5.8	6.0
Total	...	6.0	3.5	4.6	4.7

Sources: Ghana-MLG 1992, based on population census reports, and the "medium" growth rate predictions for 1995 and 2000.

Notes: Information is provided for greater Accra's three districts. Some of the most rural areas of Ga District were excluded from the survey sampling frame.

[a] Projections.

Table 2—Poverty levels in Ghana

Area	1987–88		1989		1992–93	
	Head count[a]	Proportion[b]	Head count[a]	Proportion[b]	Head count[a]	Proportion[b]
	(percent)					
Accra	8.5	1.9	21.9	4.7	23.0	6.0
Other urban	33.4	23.5	35.1	19.5	27.7	22.0
Rural coastal	37.7	14.4	44.6	16.5	28.6	12.9
Rural forest	38.1	30.3	41.9	30.3	33.0	31.0
Rural savannah	49.4	30.0	54.8	29.0	38.3	28.1
Ghana	36.9	100.0	41.8	100.0	31.4	100.0

Source: World Bank 1995.
[a]Share of population below the poverty line in region.
[b]Accra's share of national poverty.

Poverty in Accra

The proportion of the city's population living in poverty has grown rapidly. Between 1987 and 1993, the proportion living below the poverty line increased from 8.5 percent to 23 percent (Coulomb and McKay 1995; World Bank 1995)[2]. In fact, poverty in Accra increased when poverty in some other parts of the country was decreasing (Table 2).[3] Registered unemployment rose by 20 percent during the same period (ISSER 1995), with people unable to find wage employment crowding into the relatively limited range of self-employment alternatives in the city's informal economy. In 1980 the ratio of informal sector workers to formal sector workers in Ghana was two to one. By 1990 the ratio was five to one.

The flourishing informal sector, which is dominated by various forms of petty trading, has become a major public policy problem for city authorities. Informal traders cause congestion on major streets and, because of their mobility, are difficult to tax (Aforo 1997). The most recent figures continue to show extremely slow growth in formal employment opportunities, so that displaced workers (both skilled and unskilled) continue to rely heavily on the informal economy (Sawyerr and Bortei-Doku Aryeetey 1997).

The data in Table 2 for 1987–93 are drawn from three rounds of the Ghana Living Standards Survey (GLSS). But the results of the first round of the GLSS, which date from 1987–88, have been analyzed and distributed much more widely than the results of later rounds and have provided the basis of much recent policymaking (GLSS 1988; GLSS 1989; GLSS 1993). Another prominent study based on the first

[2] The World Bank poverty line is calculated as two-thirds of mean income, as measured by expenditures.

[3] Several analysts have noted that the increase in urban poverty between 1987/88 and1989 (shown in Table 2), is too marked to be an accurate reflection of actual changes (World Bank 1995). While this discrepancy may represent a measurement or methodological problem, World Bank researchers were unable to find an explanation.

round of GLSS, noted that "poverty in Ghana is an overwhelmingly rural phenomenon . . . " (Boateng et al. 1992, 56). In part because of the emphasis on rural poverty, urban poverty, food insecurity, and malnutrition have tended to receive relatively little attention from policymakers in Ghana.

A recent World Bank (1995) report on poverty in Ghana finds the decline in living standards in Accra worrisome in light of the country's economic recovery and growth. The evidence on income inequality is mixed, however. The World Bank study concludes that real mean income in Accra fell between 1987 and 1992 but that income distribution narrowed, suggesting a reduction in income inequality. The decline in living standards was greatest among the middle class, but the poverty gap widened in Accra in 1992 (World Bank 1995). Although the real average monthly earnings per employed worker climbed by 20 percent in 1987–92, the proportion of the population living below the poverty line increased from less than 1 in 10 to almost 1 in 4 (ISSER 1995; World Bank 1995). The Gini coefficient for income data on households in Accra was 0.43 for the 1987–88 round of the GLSS and 0.50 for the 1992 round. These facts suggest that inequality actually increased. The greater Accra area still has the lowest overall incidence of poverty of any of the regions for which data were disaggregated. However, the data also indicate both an increase in the absolute number of people in poverty in Accra and a narrowing of the rural–urban gap in terms of real income.

Goals of the Study

The Accra Urban Food and Nutrition Study aims to provide an understanding of the nature of urban poverty and the relationship between urban poverty and food insecurity (or malnutrition) in Accra. It sets up a framework for determining these relationships and offers decisionmakers policy options they can use to address the underlying causes of urban poverty. These policy options include interventions to support livelihoods, promote food and nutrition security, and create an enabling environment for community-based informal safety nets in areas where governments cannot afford to provide formal services.

Specifically, the study undertakes to

- identify ways that constraints to livelihoods, income, women's labor, and child care practices affect food and nutritional security in a major urban center in Africa;
- understand the strategies urban dwellers use to cope with poverty (including informal safety nets) and identify vulnerable groups;
- develop indicators of livelihood and food security that are appropriate for urban contexts;
- identify policies and programs to reduce urban poverty, food insecurity, and malnutrition; and
- provide high-quality information to policymakers in national and local governments, nongovernmental organizations (NGOs), and community-based organizations.

The policy recommendations are intended to complement policies and programs designed to alleviate rural poverty. The same report that brought the issue of growing urban poverty to the attention of Ghanaian policymakers notes that while rural poverty is declining, it is still at higher levels than poverty in Accra (World Bank 1995). Further, the most recent national data also show that the prevalence of malnutrition is generally lower in Accra than in the rest of Ghana (Ghana Statistical Services 1993). Clearly, alleviating both rural and urban poverty is essential to Ghana's development.

In terms of the national political economy, two facts are important to this analysis. First, given Ghana's current economic and demographic trends, the problems highlighted here will continue to worsen faster in Accra than in rural areas. Second, groups of urban dwellers already exist that are as badly off as certain rural groups in terms of the kinds of indicators this study uses—particularly for income, food security, health, and nutritional status. So, another major purpose of this study is to identify these groups and the constraints to their livelihood and welfare, in order to recommend policy and programmatic interventions that make sense in specifically urban settings. Given the constraints to resources and the likelihood that priority will continue to be given to rural development policy, policymakers must be armed with current status of urban populations and low-cost tools to identify vulnerable urban groups, to intervene to support livelihoods, to promote food and nutrition security, and to create an enabling environment for community-based informal safety nets where governments cannot afford to provide adequate formal support programs.

Creating an Analytical Framework

One aim of the study is to provide an overall framework for analyzing the linkages between livelihood security and nutritional security and factors such as income, women's labor, and child care practices. Several distinctly different conceptual literatures provide the background for this framework.

The Livelihood Security Approach

Household decisionmakers must decide how to use their limited resources to meet their minimum needs and other obligations. The livelihood security approach offers a holistic framework for assessing the resources and assets that are available, and analyzing how these are linked to the strategies that are used to reach desired outcomes. The notion of "livelihoods" as an organizing principle for the study of income and access to food and the basic welfare needs draws on Sen's (1981) tradition of analyzing entitlements. Entitlements are the legal means by which an individual or household gains access to their needs. These include exchange (most commonly labor for money), production using resources and labor, and transfers and inheritance. More recent work looks not only at sources of entitlement, but also demands made on entitlements including obligations to kin outside the immediate household, or indebtedness (Swift 1989; Davies 1996). Because people have to make choices among competing needs and limited resources, the notion of "livelihood security" has come to be a more all-embracing term for analysis of household resources, assets, production and exchange activities, needs, and consumption than "food security," even though food is almost without exception the most important consumption item.

Some analysts define livelihood security in terms of outcomes—particularly sustainable access to sufficient income (Frankenberger 1996). Chambers and Conway (1992, 6–7) define sustainable livelihoods in terms of capacities and activities:

> A livelihood comprises the capabilities, assets (stores, resources, claims and access) and activities required for means of [earning a] living: a livelihood is sustainable which can cope with and recover from stress and shocks, maintain or enhance its capabilities and assets, and provide . . . opportunities for the next generation.

Figure 1 maps out some of these relationships at the household level in a very simple way. The resources at a household's disposal comprise both human capabilities—skills, education, and the ability to work (including the availability of work as well as the health and nutritional status of workers)—and other assets such as natural resources, savings and financial resources, and the web of social relations in which members of the household engage. Decisions regarding how these resources are mobilized and allocated and the activities that result from these decisions constitute livelihood strategies. They include not only activities that directly earn income, but also the coping strategies used when normal income-generating activities fail or are inadequate for sufficient outcomes. And they include other household activities that do not generate income but are necessary for achieving welfare. The income, however much or little, resulting from these activities must then be allocated to competing demands, consumption, investment, or savings in order to achieve desired outcomes, which include the basic needs depicted in Figure 1: food security, nutrition, health, water, shelter, education, and a healthful environment. Desired outcomes also include other, less tangible variables including social relationships and participation in community activities. The outcomes achieved in one time period have a direct effect on the assets that an individual or household can utilize in the

Figure 1—Livelihood security at the household level

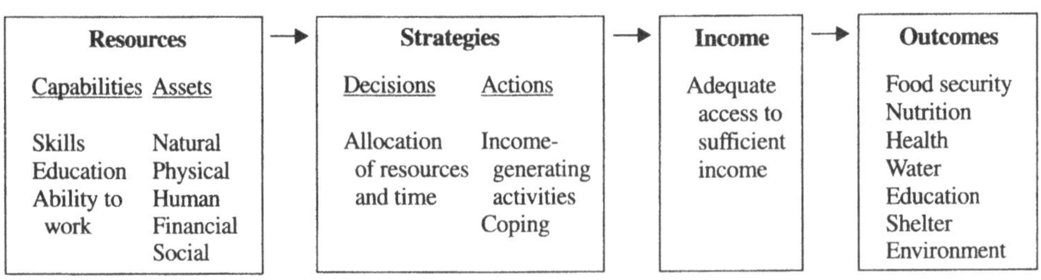

next time period: for example, sacrificing consumption to achieve improved outcomes in terms of savings or investment will result in improved financial assets but deteriorated human capabilities, and vice versa.

The assets, strategies, and outcomes at the household level must be understood in context, and the major contextual factors to consider are those that increase or decrease vulnerability—the political, economic, social, and institutional context in which the household is situated. Current status indicators—such as those listed under "outcomes" in Figure 1—describe poverty, malnutrition, poor health, and other outcomes in the current time frame. Vulnerability is a measure of the risk that one of these will occur at some point in the future. Vulnerability and poverty are not the same thing (Lipton and Maxwell 1992). People may move in and out of poverty over time; vulnerability is a major determinant of whether people actually do fall into poverty.

Vulnerability is a difficult term to define operationally. At root, vulnerability is a combination of exposure and risk and of the ability of households and individuals to cope with those risks and to recover from a shock or deterioration of current status (Chambers, 1988; Watts and Bohle, 1993). Vulnerability and the ability of an individual or household to recover from shocks is linked to the resources or assets that an individual or household holds: in general, the greater the level and diversity of assets held, the less vulnerable the household. Thus the relationships of vulnerability, assets, and livelihoods to poverty, food insecurity, and malnutrition are important to understand.

In brief, a livelihood approach helps to focus analytically on several questions: In view of known obligations and risks, how do households and individual decision-makers within households organize and manage their labor-based, income-generating activities and other forms of income and assets? What are the various means of coping with shocks: formal safety nets, kinship networks, or household-based mechanisms? How do they protect both their future ability to earn a livelihood and ensure food and nutrition security and their access to other basic necessities? This applies to both the individuals within the household and the household as a unit.These are the overarching questions addressed from a livelihoods perspective.

A Conceptual Framework for Nutritional Status

The conceptual framework for analyzing nutritional status is adapted from UNICEF (1990). Figure 2 shows the major elements of the framework . The immediate determinants of nutritional status (dietary intake, health, and care) do not differ in urban and rural contexts. But urban households may have a more difficult time than rural ones in maintaining adequate nutritional levels. Urban households are more likely to have to use cash incomes to buy food and health care, for example, and may suffer more stress from crowding and poor environmental hygiene. Women's ability to provide care is increasingly affected by the need to provide additional cash income. As demands on their time grow, women are less able to provide adequate levels of care.

Figure 2—Conceptual framework for analyzing nutritional status

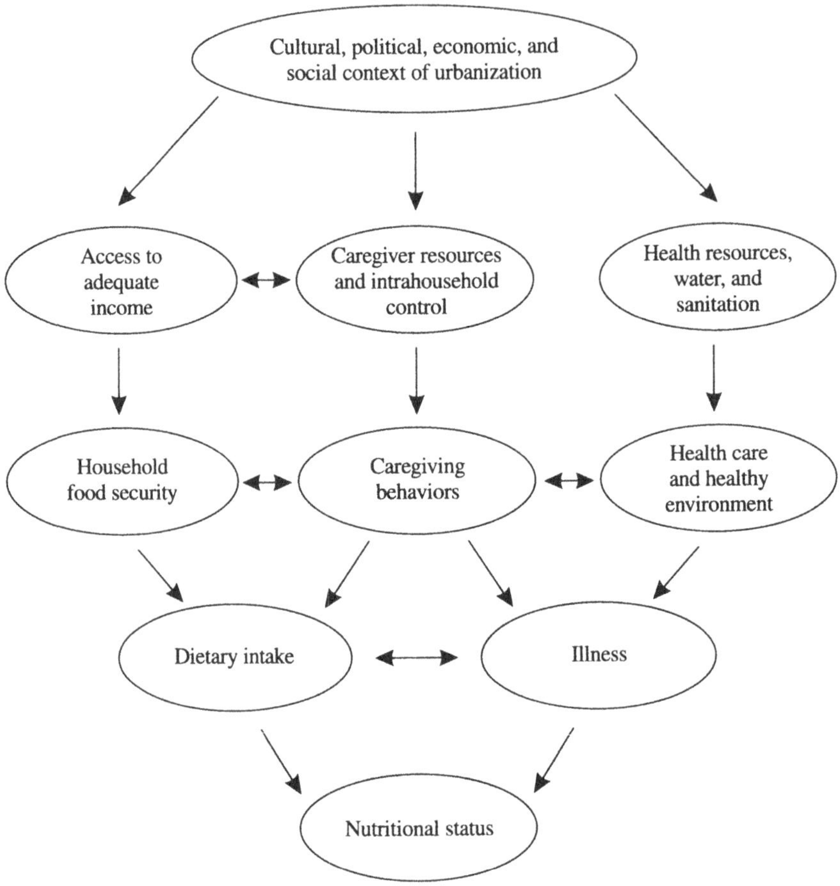

Source: Adapted form UNICEF 1990.

Care in this context is the provision (in the household and the community) of time, attention, and support to meet the physical, mental, and social needs of the growing child and other household members (ICN 1993). Even where there is poverty, food insecurity, and limited access to health care, enhanced caregiving within the household can optimize existing resources to produce good health and nutrition in young children. Recent research has suggested that care may be a particularly important determinant of good nutrition under urban conditions (Engle et al. 1997).

Six major categories of human resources for care have been identified. These include: (1) caregiver education, knowledge, and beliefs; (2) caregiver health and nutritional status; (3) mental health, lack of stress, and self-confidence of the caregiver; (4) the caregiver's autonomy and control of resources; (5) the workload and available time of the caregiver; and (6) the availability of alternate caregivers and social support from family and community (Jonsson 1995; Engle, Menon, and Haddad 1996). The household's economic resources and organizational resources at the community level interact with the human resources described above, and together will influence the set of caregiving behaviors observed within the household. Last, care is also influenced by policies and ideologies that support or undermine a household's ability to provide care, including wage policies, health care policies, and the promotion of breast-feeding.

The UNICEF conceptual framework has helped to motivate the inclusion of care as a determinant of child malnutrition; however, relatively few studies have explored the interactions between care, food security, health, and nutritional status. Part of the problem was a lack of consensus on the components of care. More recently, researchers have developed a conceptual framework for the constituents of care (Engel 1992). Once the concept of care was developed, additional research explored a set of indicators to measure care and to differentiate between care resources and care behaviors and practices. This study builds on previous research and constructs an indicator to measure care and evaluate its impact on children's nutritional status in an urban environment. The need to analyze food security, health, and nutritional status in light of the resources and behaviors affecting care is urgent. Appropriate information can give decisionmakers the tools they need to devise policies and programs to support the provision of adequate care in urban households.

Combining Livelihoods with Nutritional Status

Livelihoods—the capabilities, assets, and strategies which individuals and households bring to bear in the process of living—highlight some of the more distal determinants of nutritional status in the UNICEF framework. The UNICEF framework highlights several of the outcomes (food security and health) and some of the activities (care) that appear in the livelihood framework. The livelihood framework takes note of some of the trade-offs that households and caregivers are forced to make, both in terms of how they allocate their time and resources, among the different outcomes that can be achieved with limited income.

The analytical approach in this study, therefore, is to begin with an in-depth examination of urban livelihoods strategies, revealed by household income sources and expenditure patterns, before proceeding to a consideration of livelihood outcomes that include household food availability and distribution, health and care practices, and nutritional status.

CHAPTER 2

Design and Methodology of the Study

The study took place in four stages (Figure 3). An initial roundtable seminar in Accra brought together all parties with a stake in the outcome: researchers, city managers, policymakers, government representatives, nongovernmental organizations (NGO), program staff, community leaders and activists, and representatives of international organizations and donor agencies. The seminar's purpose was to identify information gaps that hinder the formulation of effective food and nutrition policy and programs and limit the basic understanding of urban food and nutrition security in Accra.

The second stage involved participatory rapid appraisal studies in two communities in the greater Accra area—one in a densely populated city center, the other in a rapidly growing peri-urban location. During the third and fourth stages researchers undertook a series of qualitative citywide household case studies and an integrated household survey that covered 559 households in 16 enumeration areas. Follow-up qualitative investigations helped in interpreting survey findings.

The study also investigated food production and other types of urban and peri-urban agriculture, relying partly on the household survey and partly on participatory methodology.[4] Researchers interviewed respondents, conducted feedback sessions in each enumeration area or survey site, and organized a national seminar to present results. The research design and methodology of the survey are described in detail in Annex 1 of Accra Study Team (1998).

Qualitative Data Collection

Many of the research methods used in this study were adapted from rural studies, including the participatory rural appraisal (PRA) approach and household survey methodologies. To ensure that these methods would be applicable in an urban setting, researchers devoted considerable effort to adapting and testing them in different locations in Accra (D. Maxwell 1996). An interdisciplinary research team of econ-

[4] Results of these studies are summarized in Maxwell et al. 1998.

Figure 3—Research activities, by quarter, 1996–98

Year	Quarter	Consultation	Qualitative data collection	Quantitative data collection
1996	1	• Roundtable meeting	• Key informant interviews	
	2		• PRA studies[a]	
	3		• Household case studies	• Questionnaire development
	4			• Survey training
1997	1			• Survey data collection • Data entry
	2	• Urban agriculture meeting	• Key informant interviews	
	3		• Urban agriculture studies	• Data cleaning • Data analysis
	4		• Focus groups	
1998	1	• Feedback to enumeration areas	• Focus groups • Write-up	• Data analysis • Write-up
	2	• National seminar		

[a] Participatory rural assessment.

omists, nutritionists, epidemiologists, demographers, and sociologists was recruited to carry out the testing and to incorporate and adapt various methodologies.

The first qualitative data collection activities were rapid assessments (using PRA methodologies) of two communities in the study area: an indigenous, densely populated, low-income slum area in the center of the city and a growing peri-urban community on the outskirts of the study area. The assessments were undertaken in collaboration with staff members from two local NGOs, thc local government, and representatives of the communities themselves. The results of these studies were published separately (Ga Mashie Study Team 1996; Ngleshie-Amanfro Study Team 1996).

The second qualitative activity was a series of household case studies made in a number of communities across the study area. These studies were designed to help researchers develop the survey questionnaire and hypotheses and to provide a more detailed description of the study area. The third activity was a series of focus group interviews organized around specific topics, including coping strategies, compound household relations, livelihoods, and livelihood categories. Separate reports were not issued for the case studies, focus groups, or informant interviews.

These qualitative activities allowed researchers to develop a survey instrument and hypotheses, adapt rural research methods to an urban context, and form a picture of the study area. The activities had other benefits as well. They proved invaluable in developing a definition of the term *household* that would be specific to Accra. They helped in interpreting unexpected findings and in identifying appropriate follow-up activities. They brought extreme cases (particularly of highly vulnerable groups) missed by the survey sampling strategy, to the attention of researchers. Finally, they provided researchers with an understanding of residents' perceptions of the study.

Data Collection

The basic sampling units for the survey were households with children under the age of three.[5] However, no information was available about the number of households with children in this age group in the study area. This information, therefore, had to be ascertained by conducting a complete census of the selected neighborhoods involving the enumeration of all resident households and their demographic composition.

Survey Sampling Strategy and Sample Size

The study team adopted a two-stage sampling strategy, and the Ghana Statistical Service (GSS) mapped out enumeration areas for primary sampling units in the greater Accra area. These enumeration areas were mapped in 1981–84 and had not been updated at the time of the survey, so total population estimates had to be adjusted by mean growth rates at the district level. The sampling frame included 879 urban and 33 peri-urban enumeration areas within the Accra, Ga, and Tema districts. Sixteen numeration areas were selected using a systematic sample from a random start.

The two-stage cluster sampling strategy required taking into account the design effect—the extra component of the total variance that arises because observations within clusters are more similar than observations from different clusters. Because of this homogeneity, cluster sampling requires a larger sample size than a simple random sampling. The design effect was calculated on the basis of the intercluster corrections in mean height-for-age Z-scores in previous Demographics and Health Survey data on children in Accra (GSS 1994). In order to detect statistically significant differences of 0.5 Z-scores with 90 percent power, researchers calculated the

[5] There is a growing consensus among nutritionists that the appropriate age group for measurements is children under three, not the under-five group that has often been measured. While growth curves are applicable to children under five, the risk of mortality from malnutrition decreases dramatically after age three. Because stunting may be purely a reflection of past malnutrition, interpreting stunting data accurately thus becomes difficult. This study conforms to these new trends in nutritional measurement (GSS 1994; Beaton 1993).

minimum required sample size as 36 households in 16 enumeration areas, for a total of 576 households. The same sample size was adequate to estimate the prevalence of malnutrition with a precision of plus or minus 3 percent.

No listings of households were available for the enumeration areas, so the study team conducted a census of all households within selected blocks. The final sample size was 559 households distributed among 16 primary sampling units. For many variables, however, only 556 observations were available, and this value was taken as the final sample size.

Conducting the Study

The questionnaire was pretested extensively in different areas of the city and in peri-urban areas. Table 3 shows the contents of the questionnaire, by module and respondent. A community information questionnaire was developed to collect information on infrastructure, environment, and services (or distances to services). Information was gathered for each enumeration area of the survey.

Researchers recruited a team of 25 enumerators and trained them in survey methodology and interviewing skills. The enumerators helped translate the questionnaire into the languages spoken in the study area, including English, Ga, Hausa, and

Table 3—Contents of questionnaire by module, respondent, and method

Number	Module	Respondent	Method
1	Consent form	PHM (or HHH)	Verbal consent
2	Household roster/demography	PHM (or HHH)	Recall
3	Employment and self-employment	HHH and PHM (and all economically active)	Recall
4	Adaptive strategies	HHH	Recall
5	Credit, transfers, and other income	HHH (or PHM)	Recall
6	Agriculture, livestock, and fishing	HHH (or PHM or other)	Recall
7	Food habits and coping strategies	PHM	Recall
8	Meals roster	PHM	Recall
9	Food consumption and expenditures		Recall
	a) Household consumption	PHM	
	b) Individual consumption of prepared food away from home	Specific individual	
10	Nonfood expenditures	PHM and HHH	Recall
11	Health and care	PCIC	Recall and visual analog scale
12	Hygiene spot check	Check list	Observation
13	Anthropometry	PCIC, IC, all children <5 years	Anthropometry

Source: Accra Study Team 1998.
Note: PHM = principal homemaker; HHH = head of household; PCIC = principal caregiver for the index child; IC = index child.

Twi. Five enumerators were selected for specialized training in anthropometric measurement. All were standardized to a common reference and supervised by a guest researcher who was herself standardized to an international reference.

Training for the enumerators and pretesting for the questionnaire took place during an eight-week period in late 1996. The survey was carried out between January and April 1997 (Figure 3). Questionnaires were field checked, first by the immediate supervisor and subsequently by the field manager. Supervisors made random spot checks on all enumerators each week. A double-entry system was used to minimize data entry errors, and all discrepancies were corrected by reference to the questionnaire.

Limitations of the Study

The survey sample is representative of those who live in households with children under three years of age. One child in each household in the 0–36 month age group was designated as the index child.[6] As a result, the descriptive statistics reported in this study are not necessarily representative of all households in Accra. The survey sample also did not include urban residents who do not live in households—that is, street children or the homeless population. These groups were included in the qualitative elements of this study. Other researchers have studied most of these groups (Apt Van Ham, Blavo, and Opoku 1991).

Determining how households allocate their resources was not a major objective of the study. Some individual-level and gender-disaggregated data were collected, including data on gender-specific expenditure items. But a complete intrahousehold analysis was beyond the scope of this study and should be recognized as one of its limitations. Likewise, given the emphasis on women as primary care providers, this study provides relatively little information on the role of men.

The limited number of enumeration areas suggests that the results of the survey, while statistically representative of the city, have probably not captured its extremes of wealth and poverty. Case study results, particularly among the most vulnerable groups, confirmed this observation. Interpretation of the survey results is limited by the fact that these data are cross-sectional, resulting from a single round of data collection. The survey was timed to fall between the immediate postharvest period, when food prices are traditionally at their lowest, and the rainy season, when prices are at their highest. Because of the timing, the consumption data represent an "average" picture, but the survey results do not capture seasonality. Future surveys may be able to capture seasonal differences in food and nutrition security, quantify the rate at which income-generating activities change, and determine the seasonal importance of labor migration strategies.

---

[6] If there was more than one child in the household under the age of three, the one whose first name is first in alphabetical order became the index child. All children in the survey households were measured anthropometrically, but information on feeding and care practice was only collected for the index child—one per household.

CHAPTER 3

Accra's Households and Communities

Urban areas include a diversity of peoples, and Accra is no exception. Under such circumstances, households may be organized in a number of ways, and defining the term *household* can be difficult. The classic definition of household used for survey research in Ghana involves coresidence and consumption "from a common pot." This definition applies to a portion of Accra households, particularly those in middle-class or migrant neighborhoods. However, the indigenous people of Accra, the Ga, have a unique form of household organization. For this group, with its compound households and complex living units, researchers created a new definition of household.

Ga Living Units

Despite being a small group in the overall national population, the Ga make up about one-third of the population of the city—32 percent of the sample of this study. Kilson (1974) notes that Ga men and women traditionally live in separate houses, even after marriage, and that marriage itself is a very weak institution. Men traditionally live with kinsmen from the father's side and women with kinswomen from the mother's side. In this system, children are raised in the mother's house, and male children are sent to live with their fathers around the age of 10. Households (*shia*) "are not stable groups—they are specific to particular individuals in particular social contexts" (Kilson 1974, 20). Among more educated Ga, married couples cohabit. But contemporary households in low-income indigenous areas of the city show evidence of the same pattern Kilson noted in the 1960s (Robertson 1984; Fayorsey 1995; Ga Mashie Study Team 1996). Fayorsey (1995, 92) notes, "The characteristic principle underlying Ga residential patterns is that Ga men do not live with their wives."

Many forces in the Ga community—some of them traditional, such as separate male and female residences, and others contemporary, such as high male unemployment and migration out of the community—have combined to create large compound houses in low-income indigenous communities. These households, labeled "compound matricomplexes" by Fayorsey (1995), are often headed by an elderly woman.[7]

They consist mostly of adult women and their children, although some adult men may live in a mother's residence. A typical compound household noted during one of the community studies consisted of 55 people sharing a compound of 8 rooms with a total area of around 350 square feet. The matriach, a Ga in her late sixties, described the basic composition of the compound: "I have children, and all my sisters have children, their children also have children, and our grandchildren also have delivered, and all this constitutes our household."

Most of the adult women in the compound shared the same income-generating activity—the preparation and sale of *kenkey* (the local staple food made of fermented maize dough). Both polygyny and women with children by more than one man (although never polyandry) were noted. Men as old as 40 years live in the house, but only because it is their mother's house and they have nowhere else to go. The women stated that their male children usually go to live with their fathers sometime between the ages of 8 and 15 (Ga Mashie Study Team 1996).

Income generation, consumption, and residential patterns in these households do not conform to patterns observed in households made up of nuclear families—the kind of households that predominate in Accra's migrant communities. Smaller subunits exist within these large compound houses, usually an adult woman and her dependent children. Sometimes these smaller units include the adult woman's husband or partner, who might eat with this group even if he does not live with the woman. But often the husband or partner is not considered part of the group. While coresidence does not define these smaller units, shared consumption usually does. Shared consumption usually includes not only food made and eaten at home but the allocation of money for the purchase of street foods or foods prepared outside the household.

The smaller units in compound households became the basis of the definition of a Ga household for the survey, since they were defined largely in terms of consumption and were comparable in terms of composition to households in other areas of the city. The definition therefore became *a group of people who eat from the same pot when food is prepared at home and who get money for street food from the same source.* Researchers arrived at this definition only after exploring the unique characteristics of these subunits.

First, while these households rely heavily on reciprocity and thus seem to have a built-in safety net within the compound, they are in many cases the locus of the most severe poverty in the city (Bortei-Doku Aryeetey and Aryeetey 1996). Second, overcrowding means that some people, while not accurately categorized as "homeless" in the usual sense of the word, do not have a permanent place where they sleep. They may sleep in shifts, and people who are part of a household may not sleep with

---

[7] The result of this study confirms Fayorsey's (1995) observations and has implications for understanding not only the nature of the household but also the nature of child care.

that household at all (Ga Mashie Study Team 1996; Fayorsey 1995). For this reason, coresidence does not define these households.

Third, because of the heavy reliance on street foods, consumption from a common pot alone is not an adequate definition of the household. This situation is further complicated by the fact that children in these households often eat somewhere other than with their mothers.[8] Substantial amounts of food, money, and services (such as shared childcare) are transferred among these households. Fayorsey (1995, 106) notes that

> Current urban Ga households are characterized by a group of individuals engaged in productive activities together, but they retain the fruits of their labor [individually]. Such households are characterized by exchange rather than by a pooling together of [income]. There is, however, a great deal of reciprocity. As members of the matricomplexes, urban Ga women are expected to feed and care for any child belonging to the matricomplex when the children's mothers are not around. . . .

Fourth, given the very loose attachment adult men have to these households, the proportion of households headed by women is often very high. Thus women often have considerable autonomy over their own activities, both productive and reproductive (Fayorsey 1995; Robertson 1984). Relationships between men and women in Ga society have changed gradually in the last half of the 20th century, largely because of the loss of land and the decline of traditional male livelihoods. While these changes have given women greater independence, the situation has not necessarily improved their standard of living. As has been noted, their households are among the most economically disadvantaged in the city (Bortei-Doku Aryeetey and Aryeetey 1996).

What accounts for some of the differences between this category of household and households elsewhere in Accra that conform to a more standard definition? To address this issue, researchers included questions regarding compound households, migration status, and headship into the survey questionnaire. These questions permitted researchers to analyze this category separately and to control for household type in multivariate analysis.

Characteristics of Sample Households

Tables 4 through 6 provide the basic demographic characteristics of the households in the survey sample. A total of 196 households, or 35.1 percent of the total sample, were headed by women. Though female-headed households are only slightly smaller in size than households headed by males, they have a significantly higher dependency ratio, and the head herself has significantly less formal education (Table 4). Chapter 7 provides more detailed information on women's education.

---

[8] Compound houses consisting of patrilineally related kin are also common in migrant areas of Accra, especially in areas with large concentrations of migrants from the north of Ghana.

Table 4—Descriptive characteristics of Accra households, by head of household

Characteristic	All households	Male-headed households	Female-headed households
Mean household size (persons)	5.1	5.2	4.8
	(2.3)	(2.0)	(2.8)
Mean age of head (years)	38.0	39.0	37.0
	(11.8)	(10.2)	(14.2)
Mean education level of head (years)	10.5	12.2*	7.5*
	(7.7)	(8.3)	(5.4)
Dependency ratio	1.2	1.1*	1.5*
	(0.8)	(0.7)	(1.0)

Source: Accra Study Team 1998.
Note: Numbers in parentheses are standard deviations.
*Significant at the 5 percent level.

Age and Sex Structure

The sex distribution presented in Table 5 gives an overall ratio of 76 males to 100 females. In the under-15 age group, the sex ratio closely approximates the sex ratio at birth in normal populations (106–109 males per 100 females). However, there are major differences across age groups. While the ratio of males to females is around the same in the 0–4 age group, the ratio drops to 50 per 100 in the 15–39 age group and 101 per 100 among the older age groups (40 and above). The differences are magnified still further when the sample is disaggregated into male- and female-headed households.

The relative absence of males in the households sampled is a result of the sample selection strategy and the unique structure of Ga households. The sample included

Table 5—Sex ratios by age group, by head of household

Characteristic	All		Male-headed households		Female-headed households	
	Number	Ratio	Number	Ratio	Number	Ratio
Sex ratio at age						
0–4 years	740	107	477	106	263	109
5–9 years	374	98	251	93	123	108
10–14 years	280	81	180	80	100	82
15–39 years	1,108	50	761	65	347	23
40 and older	328	101	216	243	112	12
All	2,830	76	1,885	91	945	52

Source: Accra Study Team 1998.

Table 6—Distribution of household characteristics by head of household

Characteristic	All		Male-headed households		Female-headed households	
	Number	Percent	Number	Percent	Number	Percent
Household size						
2 persons	37	6.6	...	...	37	18.9
3 persons	126	22.5	81	22.3	45	23.0
4 persons	110	19.7	80	22.0	30	15.3
5 persons	82	14.7	59	16.3	23	11.7
6 persons	75	13.4	57	15.7	18	9.2
7 or more persons	129	23.1	86	23.7	43	21.9
All	559	100.0	363	100.0	196	100.0
Household members						
Head	559	19.7	363	19.2	196	20.6
Spouse	363	12.8	358	19.0	5	0.5
Children	1,364	48.1	932	49.4	432	45.5
Parents	28	1.0	1	0.1	27	2.8
Grandchildren	208	7.3	51	2.7	157	16.6
Other relatives	283	10.0	159	8.4	124	13.2
Others	30	1.1	22	1.2	8	0.8
All	2,835	100.0	1,886	100.0	949	100.0
Type of household						
Compound	234	41.9	109	30.1	125	63.8
Nuclear	325	58.1	254	69.9	71	36.2
All	559	100.0	363	100.0	196	100.0
Migration status of head						
Indigenous	178	32.0	84	22.8	94	49.7
Not born in Accra	121	21.7	86	23.0	35	18.5
Migrant	258	46.3	198	54.2	60	31.0
All	557	100.0	368	100.0	189	100.0
Education of head						
None	56	10.0	20	5.5	36	18.4
Primary or middle school	212	57.2	173	46.7	110	66.7
Secondary school or higher	209	37.4	168	46.3	41	20.9
All	556	100.0	360	100.0	196	100.0

Source: Accra Study Team 1998.

only households with children younger than 36 months. As noted earlier, Ga children of this age tend to live with their mothers in households headed by females that often contain few adult men. This phenomenon helps to account for the very lop-sided looking sex ratios reported in Table 5.

The Size and Makeup of Households

In the Accra community, households headed by males are on average larger than households headed by females (Table 6). Overall, some 18.9 percent of households with female heads are two-person units (mother and one child). The mean size for all Accra households is 5.1 persons. The mean is 5.2 for households headed by males, however, and 4.8 for households headed by women. For all households, 81 percent of the membership consists of the head, the spouse of the married head, and their children. Relatives of the head, other than the spouse and child, make up most of the remainder (18.3 percent).

Male- and female-headed households differ in several important ways. Households headed by females contain a much larger proportion of relatives and grandchildren, and nearly two-thirds of these households are located in family compounds. Female heads tend to be younger than their male counterparts. The dependency ratio for female-headed households is also higher. The overall dependency ratio is 1.2, suggesting that there are about 120 "dependents" for each 100 people of economically productive age.[9] For female-headed households, the ratio is quite large—nearly 1.5—while for male-headed households, it is only 1.1. This demographic characteristic has important implications for both income and consumption in female-headed households. Several of the characteristics of female-headed households, particularly the low-level of education of the heads and the high dependency ratios, limit their economic opportunities and increase their vulnerability, as subsequent chapters will make clear.

Migration Status and Place of Origin

Migrant households make up a significant proportion of the total sample. Some 46.3 percent of household heads in the sample have migrated to the city within their lifetimes (Table 6). Of the remainder, 32 percent are indigenous to Accra, while 21.7 percent are not indigenous but were born in Accra. Only a relatively small number have recently migrated to the city (Table 7). The proportions of migrant households headed by males and females roughly mirror the proportions in the total sample, but only for recent migrants. Among older migrant households, the proportion of female-headed households is lower. Questions about ethnic origin were confined to the mother or primary caregiver of index children (Table 7).

Housing: Ownership and Facilities

Only 10 percent of households own their houses, while 39 percent reside in family compounds and 47 percent rented homes.[10] The remaining 4 percent engage in squatting and "perching." (This group is composed primarily of new migrants who lodge with family members, supposedly temporarily). The majority of homes (71 per-

---

[9] The dependency ratio is defined as the number of household members between 0 and 14 years and over 60 divided by the number of household members between 15 and 59.

[10] The difference between owning housing in and residing in a family compound is that ownership implies the ability to sell. Rent-free residence conveys no such right.

Table 7—Characteristics of migrant households (by longevity in Accra)

Characteristic	0–5 years in Accra	6–10 years in Accra	More than 10 years
Headship			
Male	18	34	146
Female	9	11	40
Ethnic origin (mother or primary caregiver)			
Ga/Adangbe	2	1	21
Ashanti/Akan	14	26	71
Ewe	8	12	60
Other	3	6	34
Total	27	45	186

Source: Accra Study Team 1998.
Note: 186 households.

cent) are made of concrete, brick, or stone. Toilet facilities are mainly public latrines (54 percent) and private pit latrines (20 percent). Ten percent of households have flush toilets, and 16 percent do not have access to any toilets at all (that is, household members use empty lots and gutters as places of convenience).

Vendors and wells (54 percent) are the main sources of drinking water. Another 38 percent of households have standpipes for water in the compounds of their homes, and 7 percent have indoor piping. Public dumping is the primary waste disposal method (66 percent), followed by dumping in gutters or empty lots (that is, indiscriminate waste disposal) (14 percent), household collection (12 percent), and burying or burning in the compounds of homes (8 percent).

Characteristics of Communities

Respondents in the sample rely heavily on community services and infrastructure (Table 8). At least some proportion of the population relies on public toilets in 14 of the 16 enumeration areas. One high-income neighborhood and one very low-income neighborhood do not have any public toilet facilities. The cost of using public toilets is not high, ranging from 20 cedis (₡) (one U.S. cent) to ₡80, but individuals may have to wait in a queue at peak-use hours.[11] The longest wait reported in the survey was 5 minutes, but in the community studies that preceded the survey, waits of 15 to 20 minutes were reported as common at peak-use times in the most densely populated areas. The hygiene of public toilets is poor throughout the city. Because of the cost, waiting time, and unhygienic conditions, some people choose not to

[11] The exchange rate during the survey was ₡1,950 = US$1.00.

Table 8—Services and infrastructure by enumeration area grouping

Enumeration area grouping	Number of enumerator areas	Number of public toilets within a 10-minute walk	Cost of a bucket of water	Distance to government polyclinic
			(cedis)	(kilometers)
Income quartile[a]				
1	4	1.5	79	3.0
2	4	2.5	23	0.8
3	4	2.0	36	0.8
4	3	2.3	30	2.3
Population density				
Low	1	2.0	200	0.5
Medium	3	1.0	35	2.8
High	11	2.4	30	1.5
Predominant population				
Indigenous	5	2.0	34	1.4
Mixed	5	2.2	62	1.6
Migrant	5	2.0	31	2.0
Entire sample	15	2.1	42	1.7

Source: Accra Study Team 1998.

Note: Information for one enumeration area, an upper-income quartile residential estate, is not included in this table, because much of it was not applicable. The area does not have public toilets, nor is water sold by the bucket. Refuse is regularly removed, and the nearest government polyclinic is roughly 4 kilometers away.

[a] Quartiles are based on median household income for the entire enumeration area.

use public facilities and defecate in the open. This phenomenon was reported in 9 of 16 enumeration areas.

Refuse was removed regularly in only about half the enumeration areas, and in all cases, the municipality or local authority was responsible for collecting and disposing of the refuse. Indiscriminate dumping of solid waste was noted in 12 enumeration areas. The surface drains were clogged with solid waste and other refuse in 8 locations. Even though the survey was carried out during the dry season, when Accra experiences only minor showers, researchers noted stagnant standing surface water in 9 enumeration areas.

Piped water was available in all except the peri-urban location. There, people either had to rely on rain or well water or have water brought from Accra by tanker. Even though piped water was available in other areas, its cost varied from as low as ₵20 per bucket to as much as ₵100 per bucket. The cost in the peri-urban area was ₵200 per bucket. The distance to a government clinic varied from a few hundred meters to 7 kilometers.

In general, low-income, high-density neighborhoods have poorer services and infrastructure than neighborhoods with higher incomes, but the pattern is highly variable (Table 8). For the two middle-income quartiles, infrastructure and the provision of services (as well as median income) vary little. The cost of water is skewed strongly by the high price in the peri-urban enumeration area, where no pipe-borne water is available because the area is so remote. Discounting this one area makes the cost of water much more homogeneous across all categories. And while there are more public toilets in low-income, high-density neighborhoods, the population relying on these facilities is much larger.

These are the conditions that residents of these areas of Accra face every day. The next chapter shows how they conduct their lives under these conditions.

CHAPTER 4

Urban Livelihoods: Activities, Income, Shocks, and Coping

Livelihoods in African cities no longer revolve primarily around wage-earning jobs in the formal or government and parastatal sectors of the economy. Increasingly people earn their living from informal wage labor or self-employment (ILO 1990a; 1990b). Livelihoods in Accra are limited to a fairly narrow range of activities, but these activities may be combined in complex ways and are sometimes short lived. For this reason, characterizing livelihood "systems" at the household level can be difficult, except with reference to the primary activity of the main income earner.

The livelihoods described in this study are largely labor based. While labor is undoubtedly the most important livelihood asset, several factors enhance its usefulness: education and skills, health and the ability to work, and social relations. Other demands on labor, particularly the domestic duties of women, force a trade-off between the amount of time that can be devoted to income-generating activities and the time required for other responsibilities. Reciprocal exchange (of cash and in-kind goods and services) plays an important role in supplementing and even replacing labor-based income-generating activities. Other social relations (the extended family, social networks, and so forth), play important roles, both in finding and maintaining employment and in coping with crises.

The economic crisis of the 1970s and structural adjustment policies in the 1980s have steadily eroded real income from wage labor and made finding wage employment difficult (Alderman and Shively 1996). The decline in real urban wages remained roughly the same from 1977 to 1983 in the formal private, public, and informal sectors. But wages rebounded more quickly in the formal and public sectors once structural reforms began in 1983. Informal sector wages and returns to self-employment increased briefly in the late 1980s, then dropped again in real terms in the early 1990s (Sarris 1993). Low financial assets and a lack of access to credit also limit the self-employment opportunities and small business activities. Households and individuals have responded by diversifying their income sources as much as possible (Bortei-Doku Aryeetey and Aryeetey 1996; Brydon and Legge 1996; Ga

Table 9—Employment status, individuals over the age of 10

Employment status	Male	Female	Total
Employed			
Number	398	508	906
Percent	61.4	48.2	53.3
Unemployed			
Number	55	244	299
Percent	8.5	23.2	17.6
Apprentices			
Number	22	49	71
Percent	3.4	4.7	4.2
Retired			
Number	7	21	28
Percent	1.1	2.0	1.6
Students			
Number	163	191	354
Percent	25.2	18.1	20.8
Homemakers			
Number	3	40	43
Percent	0.5	3.8	2.5
Total			
Number	648	1,053	1,701
Percent of total	38.1	61.9	100.0

Source: Accra Study Team 1998.

Mashie Study Team 1996; Ngleshie-Amanfro Study Team 1996). The range of possibilities is limited—petty trading, street food preparation, and casual labor make up the majority of the options, and competition is stiff (Ga Mashie Study Team 1996). Some people have resorted to temporary migration in search of work or trade opportunities (Tabatabai 1988).

This chapter presents evidence on labor-based, income-generating activities, total household income and income diversification, potential shocks to livelihoods, safety nets (and the lack of them), and coping strategies—especially the critical role of reciprocal exchange, remittances, and informal credit. The information gives an overall view of the livelihoods of Accra's residents—and the threats and constraints that affect people's ability to earn a living.

Labor-Based Livelihoods

Labor-based, income-generating activities are the most important source of income in the sample, particularly for poorer groups in Accra. Among all individuals over the age of 10 years in the survey sample, 53.3 percent are employed in the sense that they are engaged in a labor-based, income-generating activity (Table 9). Nearly half of all women in the sample and over 60 percent of all men in the sample fall into

Table 10—Labor classification categories

Categories	Definition
1. Protected wage labor	Cash wage work, with wages paid regularly and protected by legislation; employees are not subject to summary dismissal—that is, they are protected by a civil service appointment or by trade union representation.
2. Unprotected wage labor	Cash wage work, with wages paid regularly, but with no job security, no legal protection, and no union representation; may include piece-rate labor.[a]
3. Self-employed (productive)	Self-employment, but with the self-employed person owning capital, and producing something in the process of earning a living, or hiring or employing other persons, including family members.
4. Self-employed (marginal)	Self-employment, but with the self-employed person owning no capital, other than the stock of items for sale and working alone, without hiring other people.[b]
5. Nonpaid worker	Workers who help in someone else's enterprise but do not receive cash payment for it.

[a] Based on Harriss, Kannan, and Rodgers (1990). In that study, several categories distinguished differences in unprotected wage labor. This category was considered as a single entity for this study.
[b] In the Accra study, this category was confined to petty traders—mainly street vendors (women) and hawkers (men)—the largest category of self-employment reported.

this category. Of the remainder, 20 percent are students, small proportions are homemakers, apprentices, or retirees, and 17.6 percent reported being unemployed.[12]

The analysis of urban labor has often been based on classification schemes that do not capture the diversity of actual labor categories. Much of the analysis of urban labor in the late 1980s and 1990s has revolved around the "casualization" of labor and has focused particularly on the effects of global economic restructuring and the policy impacts of structural adjustment (Mingione 1991; ILO 1990b). A landmark study of urban labor markets (Harriss, Kannan, and Rodgers 1990) noted the importance of three factors: protection, regularity, and autonomy. That study developed a set of labor categories to analyze labor-based livelihood strategies in urban areas. These categories were adapted to analyze labor strategies in Accra (Table 10).

Men's and women's income-generating activities differ markedly (Tables 11 and 12). Almost 60 percent of men's primary income-generating strategies involve wage labor, whereas almost 80 percent of women's primary strategies involve self-employment. Men are three times as likely to have a protected wage job. More than two-thirds of women's income-generating activities involve petty trading and the preparation and sales of street food, while men's activities are more heavily concentrated in skilled and unskilled labor, clerical, and professional categories. There is one similarity, however: men and women are equally likely to be engaged in some kind of productive self-employment.

[12] The unemployed have no income-earning activity but are actively seeking one.

Table 11—All reported jobs, by category and sex of worker

Job category		Sex		Total
		Male	Female	
Agriculture/fishing	Number	46	15	61
	Percent	9.9	2.6	5.8
Petty trading	Number	26	273	299
	Percent	5.6	46.7	28.5
Street food preparation/vending	Number	2	118	120
	Percent	0.4	20.2	11.5
Small/large business[a]	Number	57	45	102
	Percent	12.3	7.7	9.7
Skilled labor	Number	166	51	217
	Percent	35.8	8.7	20.7
Unskilled/casual labor	Number	79	36	115
	Percent	17.0	6.2	11.0
Clerical/professional	Number	76	38	114
	Percent	16.4	6.5	10.9
Other	Number	12	8	20
	Percent	2.6	1.4	1.9
Total	Number	464	584	1,048
	Percent of total	44.3	55.7	100.0

Source: Accra Study Team 1998.
[a] Only nine individuals are engaged in large-scale business.

Table 12—Labor classification of primary income-generating activity, by sex

Labor classification		Sex		Total
		Male	Female	
Protected wage labor	Number	73	29	102
	Percent	15.7	5.0	9.7
Unprotected wage labor	Number	194	77	271
	Percent	41.8	13.2	25.9
Self-employed/marginal	Number	24	264	288
	Percent	5.2	45.2	27.5
Self-employed/productive	Number	169	199	368
	Percent	36.4	34.1	35.1
Unpaid labor	Number	4	15	19
	Percent	0.9	2.6	1.8
Total	Number	464	584	1,048
	Percent of total	44.3	55.7	100.0

Source: Accra Study Team 1998.

Data from Table 13 can be used to calculate the proportions of people engaged in informal and formal work, providing a means of verifying the growing trend toward informal sector employment noted in Chapter 1.[13] The calculations assume that large-scale businesses fall in the formal sector and small-scale businesses in the informal sector, so that the ratio of informal to formal workers in this sample is roughly seven to one.[14] Thus the study confirms the trend toward informal economic activities noted in Chapter 1.

Urban and Peri-Urban Agricultural Livelihoods

Much of the recent literature on food and livelihood security in African cities and the determinants of urban malnutrition has been concerned with the question of urban agriculture (Smit, Nasr, and Ratta 1996; Maxwell 1995; Mougeot 1994; Rogerson 1993; Sawio 1993). This literature notes that surprisingly high proportions of urban populations—20 to 50 percent in some cases—engage in farming and keep livestock in the city. Women do most of this agricultural work and receive most of the financial benefits from it (Sawio 1993; Freeman 1991). Recent research in African cities has shown a positive association between urban farming and both household food security (Mwangi 1995) and the nutritional status of preschool children (Maxwell, Levin, and Csete 1999).

In Accra itself, fewer than 6 percent of individuals (or about 15 percent of households) engage in any kind of agricultural production. When they do, they generally keep a few animals as a form of liquefiable assets, not for subsistence consumption or to provide a regular flow of cash income. While both men and women keep livestock, men dominate most other forms of farming in Accra. Urban production is responsible for a substantial proportion of the city's fresh vegetables, but it is mainly the wealthier classes that benefit from this production (CENCOSAD 1994).[15]

In the peri-urban area, a much higher proportion of the population depends on agriculture (Ngleshie-Amanfro Study Team 1996; Maxwell et al. 1998). But the

---

[13] The term *informal sector* is used here only as a general descriptive term, not as an analytical category. Much debate has gone into the definition of the informal sector or economy. Most of the resulting definitions revolve around the extent to which the state is able to tax and regulate such activities (ILO 1972; Leys 1975; O'Connor 1983; Portes, Castells, and Benton 1989). In the late 1980s and early 1990s, many of these activities eluded regulation, and some of them still do. But regulation and taxation do little to improve working conditions, protect labor, help enterprises grow and become sustainable, or improve access to production credit—other defining characteristics. For the purposes of this study, labor categories will be analyzed according to the classification scheme in Table 10 and without reference to any formal definition of the informal economy.

[14] In 1980 the ratio was two to one, and by 1990 it was five to one (ISSER 1995). This ratio was calculated by taking all the labor in the protected wage class, large-scale business as well as persons self-employed in clerical and professional work, and considering this group as formal sector labor, or the denominator of the above ratio. Everyone else was counted in the numerator. However, this somewhat arbitrary designation of one classification to the formal sector and others to the informal sector points out the deficiency of using the informal sector as an analytical category.

[15] For a more complete picture of urban agriculture in Accra, see Armar-Klemesu and Maxwell (1998). For a detailed analysis of the impact of urbanization on peri-urban agriculture, see Maxwell et al. (1998).

Table 13—Job category, by labor classification

Job category		Protected wage labor	Unprotected wage labor	Self-employed marginal	Self-employed productive	Unpaid	Total
Agriculture/fishing	Number	...	8	...	51	2	61
	Percent	...	3.0	...	13.9	10.2	5.8
Petty trading	Number	...	10	287	...	1	298
	Percent	...	3.7	100.0	...	5.0	28.4
Street food preparation/vending	Number	...	18	...	97	5	120
	Percent	...	6.6	...	26.4	25.0	11.5
Small/large business	Number	...	11	...	86	5	102
	Percent	...	4.1	...	23.4	25.0	9.7
Skilled labor	Number	28	102	...	85	3	218
	Percent	27.5	37.6	...	23.1	15.0	20.8
Unskilled labor	Number	23	63	...	27	2	115
	Percent	22.5	23.2	...	7.3	10.0	11.0
Clerical/professional	Number	49	53	...	11	1	114
	Percent	48.0	19.6	...	3.0	5.0	10.9
Other	Number	2	6	...	11	1	20
	Percent	2.0	2.2	...	3.0	5.0	1.9
Total	Number	102	271	287	368	20	1,048
	Percent of total	9.7	25.9	27.4	35.1	1.9	100.0

Source: Accra Study Team 1998.
Note: Leaders indicate a nil or negligible amount.

amount of land available for farming is rapidly being lost as the city expands. Some 2,000 to 3,000 hectares are lost each year in the Ga District alone (Larbi 1995). The destruction of large swathes of land in the Ga District, where sand and stone are mined for construction, further reduces available farmland in Accra. The authorities condone some of this sand mining and quarrying because it provides employment, at least in the short term. However, in the long term, it destroys the resource base of the dominant livelihood in peri-urban areas (Maxwell et al. 1998). While women and men are equally likely to lose land for agricultural production as a result of this process, women have fewer livelihood alternatives and thus are more likely to lose their primary income source when farmland is destroyed.

Multiple Income-Generating Activities

Qualitative and case study findings emphasize the importance of diversifying income sources at both the individual and household level in order to reduce risk in the urban economic environment. A relatively small proportion of individuals in the survey sample had engaged in multiple income-generating activities in the 30 days prior to the survey. A total of 124 individuals had engaged in at least two income-generating activities, and 10 had engaged in three such activities. Approximately the same number of men and women engaged in secondary activities, but the small group engaging in three activities was mostly women.

However, these findings include only activities from the 30 days prior to the survey. Qualitative information from case studies shows that an individual may engage in as many as seven or eight different income-generating activities a year. In general individuals pursue wage labor strategies when possible but engage in petty trading or other activities when circumstances permit (or require) it. Young single men are most likely to engage in multiple income-generating activities throughout the year, probably because they have the flexibility to be able to exploit multiple opportunities. Women with children have a much more difficult time pursuing such a strategy.

Despite their attempts to diversify income sources, individuals had only limited success in doing so within the last 30 days. Again, however, these data reflect only a 30-day recall, and qualitative evidence indicates greater diversification over a longer period. Further, these activities are not the only source of income.

At the household level, there is more evidence of multiple income-generating activities, and multiple activities at this level are more important to income diversification and protection against the risk of losing an income source. Roughly two-thirds of households in the sample reported that members had engaged in at least two types of income-generating activities in the previous 30 days.

In 37 households, no members had engaged in any income-generating activities in the recall period, and virtually all of these (33) were female-headed households. While this finding could be interpreted as an indication of extremely dire circumstances in other places, in Accra it is partially a result of the household structure of indigenous communities. The majority (22) of these households are headed by women indigenous to Accra, and their main source of income is through remittances, not labor. A complete reliance on remittance income, while not necessarily an indicator of poverty, is certainly an indicator of income vulnerability, given the high incidence of unemployment among men in the indigenous communities and the sometimes erratic support they are able to provide (Ga Mashie Study Team 1996). In about three-quarters of households, however, a woman is engaged in at least one of the income-generating, labor-based activities.

The average number of income-generating activities per household for the whole sample is 1.87 (Table 14). Female-headed households have a significantly lower number of income-generating activities (1.49) than male-headed households (2.08). Male-headed households utilize the labor they have more completely than female-headed households. Migrant households have a significantly higher number of income-generating activities than indigenous households.

Livelihoods under Threat

Livelihoods in the greater Accra area have been under pressure from various sources. First, the traditional livelihoods of the indigenous people—farming and fishing—have been in decline for years as the city expands into farmland and motorized trawler fleets from Tema deplete coastal fish stocks. In peri-urban areas, agriculture is declining rapidly owing to the competition for land use mentioned earlier and to environmental degradation and climatic changes (Ngleshie-Amanfro Study Team 1996).

Second, macroeconomic policies have affected urban livelihoods in several ways. Since the late 1980s, the redeployment of civil servants has put 60,000 middle-income government employees—and an unspecified number in the parastatal sector—out of work.[16] Not all of these redeployments have been in Accra, and not all those who lived in Accra at the time they were redeployed stayed there. But this group is still believed to be large in the city (Bortei-Doku Aryeetey and Aryeetey 1996). The sustained high rate of inflation—the result of policy failure—makes access to formal credit difficult. Lack of credit in turn constrains the development and growth of the small enterprises on which the vast majority of Accra's residents depend (ISSER 1997). Presurvey focus groups repeatedly mentioned lack of access to credit as a major constraint to livelihood activities but reported widespread use of informal credit.

Third, rapid population growth (particularly the migration of people of economically active ages) has meant that the number of people seeking jobs is expanding much faster than growth in the labor market. As a result, people have few options

---

[16] *Redeployment* means involuntary retirements and layoffs in the civil service or parastatals. The redeployment exercise finally came to an end in early 1998.

Table 14—Multiple income-generating activities at household level: Means and standard deviations by category of household

Category	Total number of households	Total number per household		Number to support one household member		Labor utilization	
		Mean	Standard deviation	Mean	Standard deviation	Mean	Standard deviation
Sex of household head							
Female	196	1.49[a]	0.96	0.34	0.22	0.64[a]	0.51
Male	363	2.08[a]	1.23	0.43	0.26	0.75[a]	0.41
Migration status of household head							
Indigenous	178	1.49[a]	0.98	0.38	0.27	0.68	0.49
Not indigenous/born in Accra	121	1.87[a]	1.05	0.42	0.22	0.74	0.42
Migrant	258	2.13[a]	1.14	0.41	0.22	0.71	0.42
Household lives in family/compound house							
Yes	234	1.58	1.08	0.38	0.25	0.68	0.47
No	324	2.08	1.09	0.42	0.22	0.73	0.43
Whole sample	559	1.87	1.10	0.40	0.24	0.71	0.45

Source: Accra Study Team 1998.

[a] Statistically significant difference, $p < 0.05$ (t-test for two-group comparison, one-way ANOVA for three-group comparison).

other than the limited livelihoods offered by the informal sector. This rapid growth in informal livelihoods is a double-edged sword. On the one hand, the rapid growth of the informal economy—estimated at 5.5 percent per year in the late 1980s and early 1990s—is a sign of its strength (Baah-Nuakoh 1996). On the other hand, while the number of people engaged in these activities may have grown at this rate, little evidence exists to show that the markets these activities serve have also grown. This asymmetry has reduced profit margins in the informal economy and forced many entrepreneurs to scale down their enterprises (Norton et al. 1995; Ga Mashie Study Team 1996).

Fourth, physical crowding has led to problems with the city government, which tries to keep streets and sidewalks in the downtown area clear of informal traders, removing traders forcibly if necessary. Petty street traders risk losing their stock—which often constitutes their entire working capital—if attacked by the municpal task force. These operations by the municipal task force—known by the vernacular as *abaiee* are not a daily occurrence but are frequent enough to constitute a real threat to informal trading, one of the most common livelihoods in the city, especially in the central business district (Ga Mashie Study Team 1996). The threat has prompted the formation of associations to protect the interests of informal traders, and some reforms have been implemented. The city has also constructed some new markets on the outskirts of Accra in an attempt to lure petty traders out of the congested downtown area. But many of the new markets are poorly situated in areas with few customers and now stand mostly empty.

Conflicts over the presence of more and more informal activities on the streets of the central business district of Accra—virtually all of them revolving around petty trade—have developed into one of the most urgent policy issues facing the municipal authorities. So severe has the congestion become that it has begun to block entrances to markets and shops, creating an outcry from established market traders and shop owners (Aforo 1997). The city's inability to tax petty traders, despite their proliferation on city streets, has exacerbated the situation.

Given the prevalence of petty trade, and the fact that it is the livelihood of last resort for many low-income residents (particularly women), resolving these conflicts through peaceful means is key to preserving this income source for many in Accra.[17] But the nature of the conflicting interests among the various parties involved—the city, petty traders, established market vendors and shop owners, and even the state—tends to make for a protracted problem. The city's booming population, especially among low-income groups, only makes the situation worse. And the brute force the city sometimes uses to clear the streets of traders only generates bad publicity for the authorities.

[17] The livelihoods of the lowest-income groups are the targets of municipal authorities in many cities, not just Accra. Further, this problem is just one the authorities face as they try to make the city more attractive for investment. See, for example, Becker, Jamer, and Morrison (1994) and Hardoy and Satterthwaite (1986).

Income Levels and Sources

For purposes of the study, income includes not only earned income but unearned income from the sale of property or other consumer durable goods, pensions or other government transfers, net income from gifts and remittances, lottery winnings, and savings and net borrowing or lending. Average monthly income for households in the lowest expenditure group is less than one-third of the average monthly income for households in the highest expenditure group (Table 15). Households with an unemployed head report the lowest monthly incomes. Among households whose members have classified occupations, professionals have significantly higher incomes than petty traders, street food vendors, and laborers. There are no significant differences in income levels across migration status.

Average monthly income is significantly higher for male-headed households than for female-headed households. Previous research in Ghana has shown that households headed by married women may have levels of welfare comparable to those of male-headed households and that households headed by divorced and widowed women are more disadvantaged than others (Lloyd and Gage-Brandon 1993).[18] In Accra, female-headed households are a heterogenous group in terms of family structure (Table 6), occupation (Table 11), and income level. Despite these differences, female-headed households are overrepresented in the lower-income groups. While female-headed households account for 35 percent of the total sample, they account for over 40 percent of households in the lowest income quintile and only 23 percent of the households in the highest income quintile (Levin et al. 1999).

Total monthly household income from both small- and large-scale businesses is surprisingly low. Cases in which total household income was negative during the 30-day recall period reduced these amounts (and to a lesser degree income from street vending, petty trading, and professional occupations).[19] These results may be related to two phenomena associated with collecting household income data. First, relatively wealthy households may be underreporting their income.[20] Of the 180 households with negative net returns for one or more income source, 50 percent were from the two quintiles with the highest expenditure. Average monthly household income for these 180 households was ₵171,229 per month, which is only slightly lower than the average monthly household income for the entire sample.

---

[18] Unfortunately, this study was not able to look at variations in income levels by marital status of household heads, since information on marital status was collected only for the primary caregiver of the index child. However, among caregivers, only 6.5 percent were separated, divorced, or widowed.

[19] A total of 180 households (32 percent of the total sample) had negative returns for one or more of the six sources of income listed in Table 15. Among these, 30 percent of the households were skilled laborers; 17 percent were professionals; 17 percent were petty traders; and 16 percent were engaged in small- or large-scale business. For these households, business and labor expenses were greater than income received for the past 30 days.

[20] Sensitive information, such as household income, is difficult to collect for a number of social, cultural, and economic reasons (Rozelle 1991; Christiansen 1993). In this study, some respondents did not feel comfortable revealing their true incomes.

Second, households may also report negative returns because the recall period of 30 days, which corresponds to a regular pay cycle for wage earners, does not capture the income flows for self-employed households operating home-based enterprises or engaged in petty trading or street food vending.

A third reason for negative income sources is related to the definition of household income. Unearned household income includes interhousehold transfers comprised of net transfers of gifts and net borrowing and lending. A number of households were net donors or net lenders (transfers out or the amount lent to others exceeded transfers in or the amount borrowed) and thus had negative income for the share of income from gifts, remittances, and loans.

Household Income Sources

The pattern of income by occupation group shows that while the largest share of income in most households comes from one source, it is insufficient to meet the household's total consumption requirements (Table 15). Therefore, additional income comes from a number of different sources, even among better-off households working as professionals and skilled laborers. Households engaged in activities with the lowest returns—that is, unskilled labor and petty trading—have the least diversified income sources.

Households across all expenditure groups engage in a combination of family labor and exchange-based activities (Table 15). Better-off households earn a significantly higher share of total income from self-employed productive activities than other households. These better-off households receive almost one-third of their income from self-employed productive activities, more than 20 percent from unprotected wage labor, and another 15 percent from protected wage labor. Interhousehold transfers through gifts and borrowing comprise 12–28 percent of total income, with a mean of 20 percent. Households in the lowest expenditure quintile receive the bulk of their earned income from unprotected wage labor and self-employed marginal activities (petty trading). Almost one-third of the total income of these households comes from interhousehold transfers. The unemployed receive 90 percent of their total income from gifts, remittances, and other transfers.

Indigenous households receive 30 percent of their total income from interhousehold transfers—double the amount received by migrants from that source. Female-headed households receive a significantly higher amount (43 percent) of total income from gifts, remittances, and net borrowing and lending than male-headed households (7.8 percent). Income from self-employment (predominantly petty trading and street food vending) contributes 38 percent of income for female-headed households, while male-headed households rely more heavily on wage labor.

Education is significantly and positively associated with higher per capita income levels. In households where the head of the household has completed high school or higher, the share of income from protected wage labor is significantly greater than it is in households where the head has less formal education. Households whose heads have no education or only a primary education obtain almost

Table 15—Average monthly household income and income source

Item	N	Total monthly household income	Per capita monthly income	Protected wage	Unprotected wage	Self-employed, marginal	Self-employed, productive	Rent/sales/pension/contributions	Gifts/remittances/transfers
		(cedis)[a]		(percent)					
Expenditure quintile/group									
1	114	131,434.0	21,686.7	5.7	33.9	20.9	8.1	3.1	28.4
2	111	145,992.6	27,498.9	11.2	39.7	15.9	11.7	4.7	16.8
3	112	169,336.5	32,808.3	11.3	22.7	15.9	21.7	10.0	18.6
4	111	161,328.7	38,616.7	5.7	30.2	11.4	32.8	–4.2	24.2
5	111	446,523.0	103,236.5	14.7	23.0	15.8	27.8	5.7	12.9
Occupational categories[b]									
Agriculture/fishing	13	152,053.6	30,840.5	0.0	22.4	9.5	45.7	16.4	6.0
Petty trader	95	171,587.4	31,572.3	0.5	5.8	66.3	13.3	5.6	19.3
Street food vendor	47	147,224.2	35,444.7	0.0	30.6	2.5	34.8	3.7	28.5
Business	59	130,857.3	33,690.0	0.0	20.9	–2.7	57.6	8.5	15.7
Skilled labor	149	189,595.1	40,063.6	11.7	36.8	11.4	22.7	4.0	13.3
Unskilled labor	69	139,328.0	29,650.8	15.9	58.0	3.1	–1.5	7.0	17.5
Professional	79	486,316.1	103,099.2	31.9	42.7	4.6	12.1	5.8	2.9
Occupation unclassified	7	770,690.5	118,783.1	0.0	47.0	2.2	27.6	12.4	10.9
Unemployed	37	63,373.4	20,891.9	0.0	0.0	0.0	0.0	8.5	91.5

Migrant status									
Indigenous	178	141,367.7	38,415.7	10.5	28.2	11.0	14.8	5.4	30.1
Born in Accra—not indigenous	121	222,354.0	48,030.6	6.3	33.2	13.5	25.0	4.3	17.8
Migrant	260	252,144.6	47,289.2	10.7	29.6	20.6	22.0	2.6	14.5
Gender of head of household									
Male	363	248,998.2	51,682.5	13.2	37.5	13.7	21.7	5.9	7.8
Female	196	138,977.2	31,551.8	3.1	15.8	20.2	17.9	–0.0	43.2
Education									
None	56	178,157.3	26,479.7	7.8	11.3	16.8	27.6	–2.3	38.8
Primary 1 to 6	81	136,019.8	26,497.7	1.5	40.6	30.7	9.4	2.8	14.6
Middle 1 and 3 and Islamic	72	145,102.1	32,759.3	4.4	31.9	17.4	8.0	4.6	33.7
Middle 4	158	214,505.7	44,157.2	8.4	29.3	20.1	20.0	7.3	15.0
Senior 1 and higher	190	273,984.5	62,785.9	16.9	30.9	5.7	28.1	3.0	15.4
Entire sample	559	210,422.0	44,624.1	9.7	29.9	16.0	20.3	3.9	20.2

Source: Accra Study Team 1998.

[a] US$1 = roughly 1,950 cedis at the time of the survey; text gives exchange rate as $1,950, Chapter 3.

[b] Primary job of head of household.

one-third of their income from self-employed marginal activities. The share is less than 6 percent for households with better-educated heads, however. Reciprocal exchange (gifts and remittances) makes up almost 40 percent of total income for households whose heads have low educational levels, while this figure is significantly lower for households with better-educated heads (15 percent of total per capita income).

Income Inequality

The Gini coefficient measure for income inequality for the entire sample is 0.43. This measure compares with figures of 0.43 and 0.50 for the 1987–88 and 1992 rounds of the Ghana Living Standards Survey, respectively, using only the income figures for urban Accra. (In 1992 the Gini coefficient for income throughout Ghana was 0.48.) These figures suggest that income inequality has remained fairly stable over the past decade and that income inequality is not significantly greater in Accra than in the country as a whole.

Shocks and Safety Nets

Focus groups identified the kinds of shocks to livelihoods that are common in the city. Primary among these is the loss of income from a primary income earner through death, abandonment, illness, or accident. Other shocks include unexpected family obligations (such as a funeral), job loss, failure of a small business (or an attack on it by municipal authorities), loss of access to credit, and loss of savings, especially the savings of informal lending groups (Ga Mashie Study Team 1996; Ngleshie-Amanfro Study Team 1996). Most of the shocks mentioned by focus groups tally with survey data.

Most of the safety nets developed during the post-independence era in Ghana effectively came to an end with the economic crisis of the late 1970s—especially consumer subsidies and transfers of food and money. The little that remained of these programs was scrapped in 1983 with the onset of the Economic Recovery Programme. Under these circumstances, households and individuals have had to develop their own coping strategies for dealing with financial crises. Respondents have a number of methods of dealing with shocks and income shortfalls, including transfers or informal credit and sales of assets (Table 16), and reduced spending. However, the sacrifices and trade-offs involved in these methods affect people's welfare and their productive capacity.

In the late 1980s, under pressure from various donors concerned about the severe poverty structural adjustment was causing, Ghana initiated an alternate approach to safety nets. Known as the Programme of Action to Mitigate the Social Costs of Adjustment (PAMSCAD), the program was aimed at enhancing the possibilities for self-employment among certain hard-hit segments of the population, many of them urban. Few of the formal programs begun under PAMSCAD still exist, however.

Table 16—Community, kinship, and household-level strategies

Category	Community/kinship strategies		Household/individual strategies				
	Anyone belonging to a community welfare or self help organization?	Forced to rely on interhousehold transfers in the past year?	Anyone forced to increase income-generating activities past year?	Anyone temporarily migrating for work reasons?	Income-generating activities per household	Any student forced to drop out of school in the past year?	Anyone making distress sale of personal property in the past year?
Income quintile							
1	6	48	18	9	1.91	19*	16
	(5.4)	(43.6)	(16.2)	(8.1)	(1.34)	(17.1)	(15.3)
2	8	40	15	11	1.87	10	16
	(7.2)	(36.0)	(13.5)	(9.9)	(1.07)	(9.0)	(14.4)
3	9	40	14	11	1.80	5	18
	(8.0)	(35.7)	(13.4)	(9.8)	(1.02)	(4.5)	(16.1)
4	10	40	14	15	1.83	6	15
	(9.0)	(36.0)	(12.6)	(13.5)	(1.07	(5.4)	(13.5)
5	9	43	16	17	1.96	4*	18
	(8.1)	(38.7)	(14.4)	(15.3)	(0.98)	(3.6)	(16.2)
Migration status of household head							
Indigenous	3*	80	23	22	1.49*	17	36
	(1.7)	(44.9)	(13.0)	(12.4)	(0.98)	(9.6)	(20.2)
Not indigenous/born in Accra	10	45	16	15	1.87	6	14
	(8.3)	(37.5)	(13.2)	(12.4)	(1.05)	(5.0)	(11.7)
Migrant	30*	87	39	26	2.13*	22	32
	(11.6)	(33.7)	(15.1)	(10.1)	(1.13)	(8.5)	(12.4)
Sex of household head							
Male	38	95*	58	50	2.08*	25	52
	(10.5)	(26.2)	(16.3)	(3.8)	(0.96)	(6.9)	(14.6)
Female	5	118*	20	13	1.48*	20	31
	(2.6)	(60.2)	(10.2)	(6.6)	(1.23)	(10.2)	(15.8)
Total	43	213	78	63	1.87	45	82
	(7.7)	(38.1)	(14.0)	(11.3)	(1.04)	(8.1)	(14.6)

Source: Accra Study Team 1998.
Notes: Numbers in parentheses are percentages.
* ANOVA significantly different ($p < 0.05$).

A 1996 study of poverty in Accra found that very few formal programs aimed at either poverty alleviation or reduction were operating in the city (Bortei-Doku Aryeetey and Aryeetey 1996). Researchers did find evidence of informal and kinship safety nets and observed numerous coping strategies at the household and individual levels. The qualitative studies noted a few scattered microenterprise credit and vocational training programs, but with a few exceptions these programs had tiny budgets and served a very limited number of beneficiaries. The only formal program related to food and nutrition was a nutritional rehabilitation program for severely malnourished children run by the government polyclinics in the city (Ga Mashie Study Team 1996).

This survey found no one in any household in the sample who had participated in job training programs. Seven households had received direct assistance from formal programs intended to help the destitute (these programs were usually run by religious organizations, both Christian and Muslim). Only five households included someone who had received a loan from a microenterprise credit program. These numbers are so small that it was impossible to detect any differences between beneficiaries and nonbeneficiaries.

Norton et al. (1995) report that the major constraint to the livelihoods of the urban poor in Accra is the lack of access to productive credit, a finding also confirmed by survey results and qualitative field work. These very low figures for participation in formal assistance programs are largely a reflection of the absence of such programs in Accra. The high rate of inflation in part explains the lack of microenterprise credit programs. Inflation averaged 55 percent in 1996, the year before the survey (ISSER 1997). This kind of inflation requires very high nominal interest rates, even if the interest rate is subsidized in real terms.

Coping Strategies

In the absence of formal safety nets, people rely heavily on their own strategies at the community, household, and individual levels. During times of economic stress, these strategies are likely to be the only available options.

Community and Kinship Strategies

Kinship linkages have weakened significantly over time. But they still exist among the indigenous population and can be a significant source of assistance in times of difficulty (Kilson 1974; Fayorsey 1995). Kinship linkages are also common among Accra's migrant population. But because these linkages may span considerably greater physical distances, they are often not a ready source of support in an emergency.

Urbanization has helped to weaken kinship links. One migrant woman who was supporting herself and her children by petty trade, with no support from either husband or kin, noted, "[In Accra], even close brothers may be staying together and will not even share things. One can even die of starvation and his brother will not feel obliged to help. Here, it is everybody for himself."

Numerous community organizations do exist, including occupational associations, ethnic or "hometown" associations (mostly in migrant communities), cultural troupes, and a variety of "fun clubs," drinking clubs, and other social groups. Organizations that often span the indigenous-migrant distinction include religious and occupational associations, and in some cases, labor unions and worker associations. All these organizations may, in some way, help out individuals or households in times of family crisis—particularly funerals—but they do not necessarily replace the kinship network in terms of providing emergency assistance in a financial shortfall. In the indigenous communities of the city, "town councils" help maintain cleanliness and community cohesion, although the extent to which these councils are active varies considerably.

Table 16 presents survey results on the frequency of a variety of strategies at both the community–kinship and household–individual levels. The distinction between these two kinds of strategies is based on their relationship to the household—that is, whether they rely on external resources (community–kinship) or internal resources (household–individual).[21] Participation in community welfare or self-help organizations is quite low. Subsequent focus groups revealed that this finding reflected formal membership more than informal participation, and that participation in many organizations is very informal. Nevertheless, even these data indicate a much higher rate of participation among male-headed households than among female-headed households and among migrant as opposed to indigenous households.

Household Strategies

Table 16 notes that 38.1 percent of all households reported having to rely on transfers or remittances from outside the household at some point during the previous year. In fact, survey data reveal a high degree of reliance on transfer income. Households that reported receiving assistance from kin or friends rely on this type of income for a significantly larger proportion of their total income (37.7 percent) than other households (9.4 percent). The mean proportion of income from transfers for the sample is about 20 percent.

Household strategies for coping with shocks fall into several categories:

- *Income-related strategies* include diversification, temporary migration in search of alternative income sources, and casual labor.
- *Income-pooling strategies* involve combining money at either the household or family compound level or through *susu* savings groups.[22]
- *Expenditure-reduction strategies* save money by cutting spending on consumption and purchases.

---

[21] Reliance on remittances from family members and friends is a household strategy but is listed with community and kinship strategies here because it relies on resources outside the household.

[22] *Susu* are informal groups where each member contributes a small sum each day for a month and once a month each member gets to keep the full amount collected for the day.

- *Household composition strategies* may include temporary or long-term migration, placing children in foster care, and in extreme cases, breaking up a household.
- *Food consumption or rationing strategies* use dietary changes, rationing, maternal buffering,[23] reduced consumption, and rationing through the purchase of street foods to reduce expenses.
- The *commercialization of ritual ceremonies* involves making money through events such as "outdoorings" or naming ceremonies.[24]
- *Distress sales of personal effects* bring in needed cash.

Within the previous year, 14 percent of the households in the sample had found it necessary to increase the number of their income-generating activities in order to make ends meet. Households that reported increasing income-generating activities in the previous year engaged in a significantly higher number of activities (2.57) than the remainder of the sample (1.76) and were making much better use of their labor resources. In 11.3 percent of households, people temporarily left their homes in the city and went elsewhere looking for work.

During times of severe economic stress, the most common coping mechanisms are distress sales or reductions in expenditures. Overall, nearly 15 percent of the households in the sample reported having made distress sales in the previous year. Though the money these activities generate constitute a relatively insignificant part of households' overall income, in times of stress the income is welcome. Those households reporting distress sales in the previous year obtained roughly 13 percent of their total income from this source, compared with about 2 percent of those households not reporting distress sales. The mean proportion for the entire sample is 3.8 percent.

Expenditure reduction strategies are also common. Typically, households delay large purchases (or do not make them at all), but in times of real economic stress people cut more important forms of expenditure. Food purchases, the largest and most elastic element of the household expenditures, may be the first target for reductions (Ga Mashie Study Team 1996).[25] Under more severe stress, households may cut expenditures for health care or education. In some 8.1 percent of households, a student was forced to drop out of school because of the household's inability to pay school fees during an economic crisis. Of 45 households reporting this strategy in the previous year, a total of 69 students had to drop

[23] Mothers reduce their own consumption rather than cutting their children's intake when food supplies are inadequate.

[24] Traditionally, friends and relatives give a small gift to the infant's mother at outdoorings, but this practice has become a major moneymaking scheme, particularly in Accra's indigenous communities. Many teenage girls cited this ritual as one rationale for becoming pregnant (Ga Mashie Study Team 1996). Survey data on this practice were not collected.

[25] This observation comes only from the qualitative elements of the survey. The survey data are for only one round and thus do not reflect changes in household expenditure over time. However, the perception was widespread that food expenditures are often the first to be sacrificed in a cash-flow crisis.

out of school, of whom 30 were male and 39 female. Most were the children of a household head.

The case studies showed that households employ a variety of strategies related to food consumption at times when the available food in the household is insufficient to feed all members and there is no money to buy more. In generic terms, these include dietary changes, temporary measures to increase the amount of food available, temporary measures to reduce the number of people who have to be fed, and rationing or somehow "managing" the shortfall in available food (see Chapter 5).

Individual Strategies

A variety of individual-level, income-related strategies also exist, such as taking up a sexual partner who can provide some financial support, commercial sex work (particularly in the case of women), petty crime (particularly in the case of men), and begging (particularly in the case of children, the elderly, and the disabled) (Ga Mashie Study Team 1996; Ngleshie-Amanfro Study Team 1996). Data on these practices were not collected during the survey. However, in situations where these matters could be discussed anonymously, it became clear that for certain groups under certain circumstances, these strategies were the only alternatives.

Interhousehold Transfers

In the absence of formal safety nets, interhousehold transfers are widely used to provide insurance against income fluctuations and other shocks caused by production shortfalls, unemployment, illness, and death. In fact, the most commonly mentioned strategy in Table 16 is reliance on transfers. Transfers have the potential to smooth income fluctuations, reduce inequalities in income among households, bolster investments in human capital, and ease constraints on borrowing (Cox and Jimenez 1996).

Interhousehold transfers include gifts and remittances of money and in-kind goods. They also include borrowing and lending, since the majority of credit transactions occur through informal channels—primarily among family members, friends, and casual business associates.[26] While these transfers are to some extent a daily activity, they are often a response to a financial crisis or income shortfall. They may also correspond to certain occasions, especially important passages in the life cycle—births, marriages, and funerals (Ga Mashie Study Team 1996). Overall, 83 percent of households in the survey sample reported that they had given or received a transfer in the past six months, while 79 percent reported that they had received or provided a loan.

---

[26] Gifts are transfers based on reciprocal exchange with no formal agreement that the gift will be repaid. However, reciprocity is often implicit in these gifts. Gifts are distinguished from loans, which come with a verbal or written agreement that the amount borrowed will be repaid with or without interest.

Reciprocal Exchange: Gifts and Remittances

Transfers (or gifts and remittances) are frequent exchanges of cash or food between nuclear and extended families living within Accra. Interhousehold transfers of gifts and remittances are an important source of income for some households, and the data provide several important and unexpected findings regarding these transfers. First, a strong intergenerational flow of resources from parent to child (rather than vice versa) prevails, particularly with regard to remittances sent out of the household. Second, much of the transfer activity takes place in the urban area rather than between the city and rural villages.

Most income transfers are made either within the nuclear family or between very close relatives (Table 17). Some 28.2 percent of total transfers are from husband to wife, reflecting in part the living arrangements in Ga households, noted in Chapter 3 (54 percent of these transfers between spouses occur within Ga families). This situation also reflects household organization more generally. Case study findings revealed that in Ga households husbands and wives tend to keep their incomes separate and have separate purchasing responsibilities. Couples loan or transfer money to each other regularly, whether they live together or apart (survey data capture interhousehold transfers only if husbands and wives are living apart). Income transfers between a nuclear family and very close relatives (parents, siblings) account for

Table 17—Direction of transfer flow

	Transfers received by household			Transfers given by household		
Relationship	Number of transfers	Percent of transfers	Percent of total amount transferred	Number of transfers	Percent of transfers	Percent of total amount transferred
Husband to wife	439	28.2	34.7	4	0.4	0.6
Wife to husband	...	...	...	9	0.9	0.9
Father to children	57	3.7	2.9	197	20.5	28.8
Mother to children	122	7.9	5.5	215	22.3	17.6
Brother to sibling	51	3.3	10.1	43	4.5	9.3
Sister to sibling	92	5.9	8.6	62	6.4	7.3
Son to parent	46	3.0	5.8	22	2.3	5.9
Daughter to parent	61	3.9	3.1	24	2.5	2.5
Between other relatives	253	16.3	14.1	176	18.3	14.8
Between in-laws	86	5.5	2.5	51	5.3	4.2
Between friends	346	22.3	12.5	159	16.5	8.0
Other (institution)	1	0.1	0.1	...	...	...
Totals	1,554	100.0	100.0	962	100.0	100.0
Sex of recipient/donor						
Male	188	12.1	18.0	392	40.7	60.6
Female	1,366	87.9	82.0	570	59.2	39.4
Totals	1,554	100.0	100.0	962	100.0	100.0

Source: Accra Study Team 1998.
Note: Data are for six months preceding survey.

56 percent of the total number of transfers received by the households in the survey, and they account for 70 percent of the money value of transfers.

Focus groups note that different types of transfers carry different types of social obligations. While customs vary among different cultural groups, husband-to-wife transfers place strong obligations on the wife to "please her husband." Some transfers may be reported in survey results as coming from a "husband," but it is not possible to estimate how many of the couples are actually married. Between friends, transfers tend to carry the obligation to respond in the same way if the friend who helps out is later in need. This obligation also affects natal kin, especially siblings. Finally, a major locus of transfers are ceremonies, particularly the "outdooring" of a newborn child. Gifts at these occasions tend to carry an obligation of reciprocity, but at an unspecified later time.

Respondents sent 4.8 percent of total transfers to their parents, yet 46.4 percent of respondents sent transfers to their children, accounting for almost half the money sent out of the household (Table 17). Only 7 percent of the total number of transfers received by respondents came from children, accounting for less than 10 percent of the value of incoming transfers. The majority of transfer recipients (87.9 percent) and donors (60 percent) are female.

Most transfers of goods and money take place within the city, not between urban and rural areas (Table 18). Households in Accra received 76 percent of all transfers. These households sent only 29 percent of transfers to rural areas—but 66 percent went to households in Accra or other urban areas. The notion of young wage laborers in the city remitting money to their families (especially elderly parents) in rural areas does not apply to greater Accra. First-generation migrants continue to remit substantial amounts of money and goods to rural areas. But beyond this group,

Table 18—Transfers between urban and rural areas

Direction of flows	Number of transfers	Percent of transfers	Percent of total amount transferred
Household member is recipient:			
Within Accra	1,179	76	54.8
Outside Accra	123	8	6.9
Rural to urban	150	10	6.3
Overseas remittances	87	6	32.0
Total	1,539	100	100.0
Household member is donor:			
Within Accra	421	44	40.6
Outside Accra	212	22	26.0
Urban to rural	280	29	27.0
Overseas remittances	50	5	6.4
Total	963	100	100.0

Source: Accra Study Team 1998.
Note: Data are for six months preceding survey.

Table 19—Types and uses of transfers

Transfer	Household is recipient			Household is donor		
	Number of transfers	Percent of transfers	Percent of total amount transferred	Number of transfers	Percent of transfers	Percent of total amount transferred
Type						
Cash	966	62.2	63.7	462	48.0	52.0
Food	432	27.8	20.5	346	35.9	33.1
Clothing	97	6.2	14.0	76	7.9	10.0
Medicine	6	0.4	0.2	3	0.3	0.3
Other	31	2.0	0.7	64	6.6	3.5
Unspecified	22	1.4	0.9	12	1.2	1.1
Total	1,554	100.0	100.0	963	100.0	100.0
Use						
Individual consumption	317	20.6	16.9	582	61.0	58.7
Household consumption	1,151	74.8	66.6	296	31.0	26.5
Business	24	1.6	7.2	19	2.0	2.35
Housing improvements	1	0.06	3.6	3	0.3	2.3
Health and education	23	1.5	3.2	25	2.6	7.0
Consumer durables	5	0.32	0.57	1	0.1	0.11
Other personal use and savings	17	1.1	0.92	28	2.9	2.2
Unspecified	19	1.0	1.04	9	1.0	0.81
Total	1,554	100.0		963	100.0	

Source: Accra Study Team 1998.
Note: Data are for six months preceding survey.

social relations as exemplified by reciprocal exchange are largely confined to the city itself.

Most transfers are used to meet either individual or household consumption needs (Table 19). Survey respondents reported that almost 75 percent of all transfers received by individuals living in the household go toward meeting household consumption needs.

Borrowing and Lending

Few microenterprise credit or other semiformal credit institutions operate in the city. The survey found that only 1.5 percent of loans is made through formal institutions (Table 20). Most loan transactions are informal, and over half (58.4 percent) take place between relatives or friends. Another third are made with traders or dealers who provide goods for household consumption and production. Women receive more loans than men and lend more frequently (but in smaller amounts).

Only one-third of the total loans transactions are used for business enterprises or for agricultural purposes, but these loans account for almost 60 percent of the total amount borrowed (Table 21). A number of smaller loans are used to meet individual

Table 20—Source of loan and relationship of lender to borrower

Relationship	Household is borrower			Household is lender		
	Number of loans received	Percent of loans	Percent of total borrowed	Number of loans given	Percent of loans	Percent of total loaned
Relative or friend	622	58.4	44.3	331	40.5	35.2
Commercial bank or other financial institution/business customer or associate	16	1.5	4.2	468	57.3	59.8
Susu	9	0.8	0.9	...	...	...
Nongovernmental organization	1	0.1	0.2	...	...	...
Employer	34	3.2	14.8	2	0.2	1.2
Trader or dealer	349	32.7	31.3	...	...	...
Moneylender	10	0.9	2.3	...	...	...
Other	24	2.3	2.8	15	1.8	3.9
Total	1,065	100.0	100.0	816	100.0	100.0
Sex						
Male	228	21.4	42.2	220	27.0	65.8
Female	833	78.2	57.1	592	72.5	30.9
Total	1,061	99.6[a]		812	99.5[a]	...

Source: Accra Study Team 1998.

[a] Data were missing on the sex of the borrower or lender for four observations.

Table 21—Uses of loans

Use of loan	Household is borrower			Household is lender		
	Number of loans	Percent of loans	Percent of total borrowed	Number of loans	Percent of loans	Percent of total loaned
Business enterprise or agriculture	356	33.4	57.9	222	27.2	58.9
Individual consumption	180	16.9	5.5	379	46.4	21.1
Household consumption	321	30.1	9.9	164	20.1	6.2
Housing	18	1.7	5.0	12	1.5	3.4
Education	34	3.2	3.6	15	1.8	7.2
Health care	60	5.6	2.0	11	1.3	0.6
Marriage/funeral	34	3.2	2.7	6	0.7	1.3
Consumer durables	28	2.6	10.5	...	...	...
Other personal	31	2.9	2.5	...	...	...
Total	1,062[a]	99.7[a]	100.0	809[b]	99.1[b]	98.7

Source: Accra Study Team 1998.

[a] Three missing observations.

[b] Seven missing observations.

and household consumption needs. Almost half of all loans are used to meet consumption needs, but these loans only account for 15 percent of the total amount borrowed. Given that a large proportion of credit transactions are obtained from informal sources and used to meet individual and household consumption needs, it is not surprising that 94 percent of these loans were interest free and that 61 percent were obtained without any collateral.

Susu Groups

Membership in a *susu* group is a common means of accumulating capital for either a purchase or business investment. The most common form of *susu* group is organized by a "collector." Members contribute a certain sum to the group every day. Once a month, each group member (including the collector) gets the full amount contributed that day. *Susu* groups are a means of accumulation rather than credit per se, although *susu* collectors are also a source of informal credit (Table 20). The study found that respondents often did not report *susu* income, since over the 30-day recall period used in the study contributions and money received in this way tended to balance each other out.

Susu practices are widely mistrusted in some areas of the city because of increasing tendencies on the part of *susu* collectors to abscond with money. In nearly half of all household case studies, members mentioned this problem as the reason for not participating in *susu* groups.

Clearly, a high proportion of the resources available to Accra households come from gifts, remittances, and loans. The sheer volume of the resources that are exchanged suggests that transfers and loans are an essential source of needed income and goods. Most of these resources are used for consumption purposes, however, posing a major challenge for poverty alleviation efforts. Can these informal resources be channeled toward productive investments in small enterprises and skills in order to enhance income-generating capacity in the long term? Under the current system, Accra's residents continue to face severe constraints in finding ways to improve their livelihoods.

Further Findings

Several other perceptions from the focus group discussions are worth noting. First, the majority of respondents felt that most people aim for one of two income sources in order to get enough income to survive in Accra. The first of these is ownership of a small business other than petty trading or street food vending. The second, which is much more difficult to obtain, is a job with a regular salary, even if the work does not pay all that well.

Second, while having sufficient income is important to being able to provide educational opportunities for children, education is not necessarily viewed as a major asset in terms of finding work—especially a wage-earning job. The general perception is that specific skills are more important than academic education. This belief may help explain why taking children out of school is a common expenditure-reducing strategy. Results discussed in Chapters 7 and 8 suggest that education may be valuable for more than just its potential on the job market, however.

Third, nearly all groups stressed that large families, particularly large numbers of children, are a liability. Despite the fact that roughly half of these groups were made up of women and that the evidence from the survey data showed otherwise, there was not a widespread perception that female-headed households were worse off than households headed by males.

Fourth, respondents offered a fairly common list of constraints to the livelihoods of poor individuals and households. Some of these revolved around the classic explanation for what has been called the "culture of poverty," "laziness," "irresponsibility," men with "too many girlfriends," and "poor social background." However, a second set of constraints identified through the focus groups tallies fairly closely with those derived from survey data. These constraints include a lack of salable skills, the absence of job opportunities even for those who have skills (men), lack of access to credit with which to begin small enterprises (women), poor health of the primary income earner, and conflicting demands on time. Access to credit is a major constraint to livelihoods, especially among the self-employed.

Secondary evidence confirmed other constraints that were noted in the qualitative work. First, high municipal taxes for formally registered activities tend to push people into informal (and less remunerative) activities and to keep them there. Second, the municipal authorities tend to harass small traders trying to work in the most lucrative areas of the city (the central business district). Third, too many people are crowded into too few forms of self-employment, making profit margins very low and working hours very long (Bortei-Doku Aryeetey and Aryeetey 1996). While the cross-sectional quantitative data cannot explain very much about trends in income-generating activities over time, the perception of "crowding in" to a few occupational categories and of falling incomes in those categories was very strong. Unfortunately, people see few other options.

CHAPTER 5

Household Spending, Consumption, and Food Security

How do households use their incomes to meet the basic requirements of food, shelter, water, health, and education? How successful are they in making ends meet? This chapter analyzes household expenditure patterns, focusing first on non-food items and then turning to food.

Expenditure Patterns

Estimates from the survey suggest that household incomes are substantially less than consumption (Table 22). However, household consumption expenditures are considered a more reliable indicator of permanent income, largely because they are less variable (Anand and Harris 1985). If household consumption expenditures are used as a proxy for income, the median income for the sample is approximately US$390 per person per year, roughly the average reported for all of Ghana by the World Bank (1997).

Nonfood Expenditures

Food is by far the largest item in household budgets, accounting for 54.5 percent of all expenditures (Table 23). After food, clothing is the second most important expenditure item, accounting for 8.9 percent. However, the survey was conducted near the time of several Christian and Muslim holidays, so that clothing expenditures were probably higher than normal. Miscellaneous expenses,[27] transportation, health, and utilities account for about 4–5 percent of total outlay each. Expenditures on infrastructure services (fuel and lighting, utilities, transportation, health, and education) account for 20 percent of total expenditures. The study found that in general

[27] Miscellaneous expenses include loans to others, loan repayments, remittances sent out of the household, taxes, and savings.

Table 22—Mean income and expenditures by expenditure group, occupation, migration status, education, and sex of head of household

Category	N	Total income per capita per year	Total expenditures per capita per year
		(thousands of cedis)	(thousands of cedis)
Entire sample	559	536.3	1,028.2
Expenditure group			
1	114	264.4	379.1
2	111	330.0	572.4
3	112	393.7	766.0
4	111	463.4	1,091.3
5	111	1,238.8	2,334.5
Occupational categories[a]			
Agriculture/fishing	13	370.1	757.1
Petty trader	95	378.9	851.8
Street food vendor	47	425.3	720.3
Business	59	404.3	1,344.2
Skilled labor	149	480.8	981.8
Unskilled labor	69	355.8	695.7
Professional	79	1,251.7	1,705.8
Unclassified	7	1,425.4	929.8
Unemployed	37	250.7	870.7
Migration status			
Indigenous	178	461.0	1,126.0
Born in Accra—not indigenous	121	576.4	924.8
Migrant	260	569.3	1,008.5
Education			
None	56	317.8	602.2
Primary 1 to 6	81	318.0	780.6
Middle 1 and 3 and Islamic	72	393.1	797.3
Middle 4	158	532.6	905.5
Senior 1 and higher	190	753.4	1,452.8
Gender of head of household			
Male	363	621.6	1,135.1
Female	196	378.6	830.3

Source: Accra Study Team 1998.
[a] Primary job of head of household.

women pay for fuel, clothing for themselves and children, transportation, and ceremonial gifts. Men are responsible for housing, health, and education.

The budget share for housing (inclusive of rents, repairs, and mortgage expenses) accounts for only 2 percent of total expenditures. This low figure may be explained by the fact that only 57 percent of the households paid rent, invested in housing repairs, or paid a mortgage. A majority of respondents either owned their homes (10 percent), resided in a family compound (39 percent), or squatted (4 percent), while the remaining 47 percent rented their homes. These figures suggest that

Table 23—Average share of major household expenditures

Category	Number of households	Total expenditures per capita	Food	Housing	Fuel and light	Utilities	Clothing	Nondurable goods	Durable goods	Household services
		(cedis)				(percent)				
Entire sample	559	1,028,181	54.5	2.1	3.7	4.1	8.9	3.7	1.2	0.2
			(100)	(57)	(98)	(97)	(98)	(98)	(27)	(4)
Expenditure group										
1	114	379,134	61.1	1.5	5.2	5.2	7.1	4.8	0.2	0.1
			(100)	(45)	(97)	(96)	(94)	(97)	(9)	(1)
2	111	572,411	61.4	1.6	4.8	4.8	7.7	3.7	0.5	0.0
			(100)	(55)	(97)	(97)	(98)	(97)	(17)	(0)
3	112	765,952	56.1	1.8	6.5	4.1	9.8	3.8	1.2	0.2
			(100)	(57)	(96)	(97)	(99)	(97)	(28)	(3)
4	111	1,091,259	53.4	2.0	3.1	3.4	9.6	2.8	1.4	0.2
			(100)	(61)	(98)	(97)	(100)	(100)	134)	(5)
5	111	2,334,509	40.7	3.5	2.1	3.0	10.3	3.4	2.7	0.3
			(100)	(69)	(100)	(99)	(100)	(98)	(47)	(12)
Occupational catagories[a]										
Agriculture/fishing	13	757,139	61.9	0.9	6.2	2.3	8.1	2.4	0.5	0.0
			(100)	(54)	(100)	(92)	(100)	(100)	(23)	(12)
Petty trader	95	851,763	58.8	1.4	4.1	4.1	7.0	3.6	0.3	0.2
			(100)	(52)	(98)	(97)	(98)	(96)	(17)	(5)
Street food vendor	47	720,304	67.1	0.4	4.2	4.7	6.7	4.9	0.2	0.0
			(100)	(23)	(98)	(98)	(94)	(98)	(11)	(0)
Business	59	1,344,161	47.0	2.4	2.7	3.7	10.1	3.4	2.5	0.2
			(100)	(69)	(97)	(100)	(100)	(100)	(37)	(5)

Skilled labor	149	981,787	51.7	2.2	4.0	4.0	9.8	4.1	1.6	0.1
			(100)	(70)	(98)	(97)	(100)	(99)	(32)	(3)
Unskilled labor	69	695,651	58.2	1.6	4.0	4.3	9.5	3.4	0.9	0.1
			(100)	(61)	(97)	(97)	(97)	(97/)	(23)	(1)
Professional	79	1,705,832	44.0	4.5	2.7	3.8	10.3	2.9	2.1	0.2
			(100)	(63)	(100)	(99)	(100)	(99)	(44)	(11)
Unclassified	7	929,786	56.4	1.2	3.7	2.8	11.0	2.6	0.6	1.2
			(100)	(57)	(100)	(100)	(100)	(100)	(14)	(14)
Unemployed	37	870,654	63.8	1.1	3.4	5.2	7.2	4.3	0.5	0.0
			(100)	(28)	(94)	(97)	(92)	(94)	(11)	(0)
Migration Status										
Indigenous	178	1,123,967	55.7	1.2	3.4	4.2	8.4	3.9	1.0	0.2
			(100)	(29)	(98)	(98)	(97)	(98)	(21)	(5)
Born In Accra—not indigenous	121	924,826	56.6	2.2	4.0	4.3	8.8	3.9	1.2	0.1
			(100)	(60)	(97)	(97)	(97)	(98)	(28/)	(3)
Migrant	260	1,008,463	52.8	2.6	3.8	4.0	9.3	3.4	1.4	0.1
			(100)	(76)	(98)	(98)	100)	(98)	(30)	(4)
Sex of head of household										
Male	363	1,135,100	51.5	2.6	3.7	3.9	9.7	3.3	1.7	0.2
			(100)	(70)	(99)	(98)	(99)	(98)	(21)	(5)
Female	196	830,300	60.2	1.0	3.8	4.5	7.5	4.4	0.4	0.1
			(100)	(34)	(96)	(97)	(96)	(98)	(15)	(3)

(*continued*)

Table 23—Continued

Category	Number of households	Health	Transport	Communication	Recreation	Education	Donations	Ceremonies	Alcohol and cigarettes	Miscellaneous
						(percent)				
Entire sample	559	4.5	5.0	0.2	1.6	1.8	1.5	0.8	0.9	5.3
		(73)	(80)	(14)	(40)	(62)	(60)	(54)	(33)	(84)
Expenditure group										
1	114	3.3	3.8	0.1	0.6	2.2	1.1	0.5	0.4	2.9
		(54)	(72)	(4)	(23)	(61)	(50)	(35)	(22)	(73)
2	111	3.7	3.6	0.1	0.8	1.8	1.1	0.4	1.0	3.1
		(68)	(80)	(5)	(27)	(63)	(48)	(46)	(30)	(77)
3	112	5.1	4.3	0.1	1.4	1.8	1.1	0.9	0.8	4.2
		(80)	(76)	(10)	(40)	(67)	(60)	(53)	(35)	(86)
4	111	5.5	4.3	0.3	1.7	2.0	1.6	0.9	0.9	6.9
		(79)	(82)	(19)	(42)	(64)	(68)	(66)	(28)	(89)
5	111	5.3	9.0	0.6	3.3	1.4	2.3	1.5	1.4	9.3
		(82)	(91)	(33)	(66)	(55)	(75)	(69)	(51)	(97)
Occupational categories[a]										
Agriculture/fishing	13	4.3	4.8	0.0	1.0	0.8	1.3	0.5	1.3	3.8
		(77)	(92)	(8)	(38)	(46)	(62)	(54)	(38)	(92)
Petty trader	95	6.3	3.2	0.1	0.9	1.8	0.9	0.8	0.7	5.7
		(68)	(81)	(11)	(25)	(64)	(57)	(56)	(30)	(89)
Street food vendor	47	3.4	2.4	0.0	0.4	1.2	0.7	0.3	1.0	2.5
		(68)	(70)	(0)	(15)	(49)	(43)	(45)	(32)	(68)
Business	59	4.8	7.6	0.6	2.8	1.7	1.5	1.1	0.6	7.5
		(71)	(85)	(31)	(49)	(68)	(63)	(59)	(39)	(92)

Skilled labor	149	3.8	5.8	0.2	1.9	1.7	1.7	0.7	1.0	5.7
		(76)	(85)	(11)	(42)	(64)	(60)	(48)	(36)	(89)
Unskilled labor	69	3.3	4.9	0.1	1.1	1.6	1.2	0.7	1.0	4.1
		(59)	(80)	(7)	(38)	(62)	(65)	(54)	(33)	(78)
Professional	79	5.0	6.8	0.6	2.4	3.2	2.6	1.4	1.0	6.4
		(86)	(83)	(30)	(68)	(72)	(77)	(66)	(35)	(86)
Occupation unclassified	7	3.2	4.0	0.0	3.8	1.1	1.8	0.9	2.0	4.0
		(71)	(86)	(0)	(71)	(57)	(57)	(86)	(43)	(71)
Unemployed	37	6.4	2.0	0.1	0.1	1.4	0.9	0.7	0.2	2.6
		(78)	(53)	(6)	(19)	(39)	(44)	(39)	(14)	(69)
Migration status										
Indigenous	178	5.4	5.4	0.2	1.4	1.9	1.3	0.8	0.9	4.5
		(70)	(78)	(12)	(35)	(54)	(56)	(53)	(36)	(86)
Born in Accra—not indigenous	121	4.4	3.8	0.3	1.6	1.3	1.3	0.9	0.7	4.7
		(79)	(80)	(14)	(37)	(57)	(55)	(49)	(26)	(76)
Migrant	260	4.1	5.2	0.2	1.6	2.0	1.6	0.8	0.9	6.1
		(72)	(82)	(15)	(44)	(70)	(66)	(56)	(34)	(87)
Sex of head of household										
Male	363	4.0	5.9	0.3	1.8	1.8	1.7	1.0	1.1	6.0
		(74)	(84)	(16)	(50)	(65)	(62)	(58)	(38)	(87)
Female	196	5.6	3.3	0.1	1.1	1.9	1.1	0.5	0.5	3.9
		(71)	(73)	(9)	(21)	(56)	(58)	(44)	(23)	(79)

Source: Accra Study Team 1998.
Note: Figures in parentheses are the proportion of households with nonzero consumption.
[a] Primary job of head of household.

Figure 4—Average share of total budget allocated to food, by per capita expenditure quintile

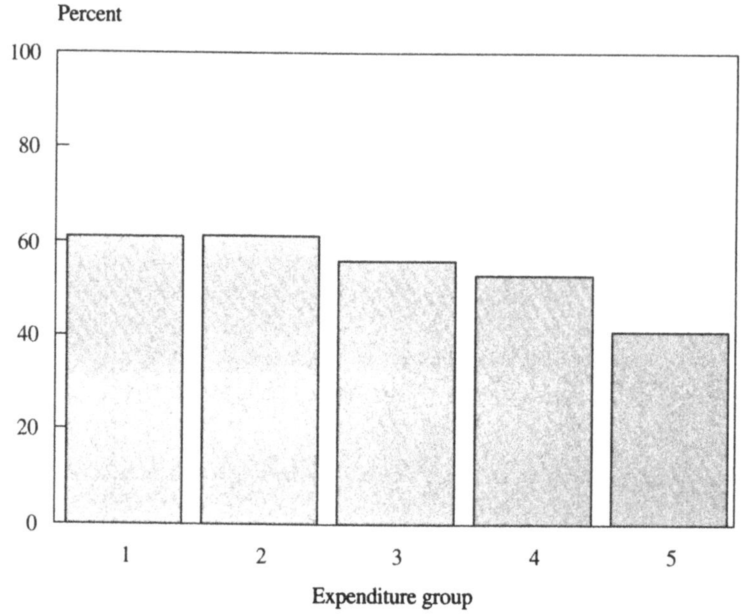

Source: Accra Study Team 1998.
Note: Group 1 is the lowest expenditure quintile; group 5 the highest.

over 40 percent of the sample save "imputed rent," or the income that would have otherwise been spent on housing costs (Moser 1996).

The budget shares for almost all nonfood categories (and positive purchases in these categories) increase with income, except for basic necessities such as fuel and lighting, utilities, and nondurable household items. Two important nonfood expenditure categories for basic services—health and education—do not fit this pattern, however. As incomes increase, so do expenditures on health. But the average share of total household expenditures allocated to education is very low for all groups.

Food Expenditures and Source of Acquisition

Overall, the most important mean household expenditure by far is food (54.5 percent of total expenditures).[28] As income increases, the percent of the budget allocated to food falls (Figure 4). This finding is consistent with the Engelian relationship between income and the percentage allocated to food (Deaton and Muellbauer

---

[28] This figure is higher than the average of 49.1 percent for Accra in the most recent GLSS (1992). The difference between the two estimates may reflect different survey methodologies used to collect household food consumption data. This survey made a special effort to collect information on food consumed away from home.

1980). For households in the lowest expenditure quintile, nearly 60 percent of total expenditures went to food, compared with only 40 percent for households in the highest quintile.

Urban food expenditure patterns in Accra are characterized by heavy dependence on purchased food commodities, including a substantial amount of street foods. For the entire sample, these purchases accounted for approximately 90 percent of total consumption, indicating a strong reliance on the market to meet consumption needs. There are no significant variations from this pattern across expenditure quintiles (Table 24).

At first glance, the figures present a rather homogeneous story of urban consumers who are almost completely dependent on the market to meet their food needs. Consumption from respondents' own production was low, accounting for less than 1 percent of total food expenditures for the whole sample, with no significant differences across quintiles. Similarly, consumption from in-kind wages was

Table 24—Mean percent of total food expenditures from different sources of acquisition

Category	Number of households	Purchased food	Own production	In-kind wages	Gifts and transfers	Food given to others
Entire sample	559	90.9	0.9	1.2	6.3	0.6
Expenditure group						
1	114	90.5	1.2	0.6	7.7	0.0
2	111	89.6	0.7	1.9	7.3	0.3
3	112	90.2	0.6	2.0	6.7	0.5
4	111	91.2	1.3	1.0	5.9	0.5
5	111	92.7	0.9	0.5	4.2	1.5
Occupational categories[a]						
Agriculture/fishing	13	78.5	7.5	4.5	8.9	0.2
Petty trader	95	89.8	0.8	0.3	7.8	1.3
Street food vendor	47	88.4	0.4	3.5	6.7	0.4
Business	59	91.4	1.0	0.7	5.8	1.1
Skilled labor	149	92.4	0.7	1.7	4.7	0.5
Unskilled labor	69	90.2	1.4	1.5	6.5	0.4
Professional	79	95.3	0.5	0.1	3.9	0.1
Unclassified	7	92.6	1.5	1.3	4.3	0.3
Unemployed	37	86.3	0.0	0.0	13.7	0.0
Migration status						
Indigenous	178	88.9	0.5	0.9	8.7	0.9
Born in Accra—not indigenous	121	91.4	1.2	0.6	6.3	0.4
Migrant	260	92.0	1.1	1.7	4.8	0.5
Sex of head of household						
Male	363	92.4	1.1	0.9	5.1	0.5
Female	196	88.1	0.6	1.6	8.7	0.8

Source: Accra Study Team 1998.
[a] Primary job of household head.

minimal, accounting for about 1 percent of total food expenditures. However, a slightly richer story emerges when the budget shares are explored by occupation groups. Only 5.8 percent of the individuals interviewed in the survey had been active in agriculture, livestock, or fishing in the previous 30 days. Most individuals earned their living through petty trade, street food vending, small- and large-scale enterprises, wage labor, or professional services in a competitive and densely populated urban environment. Even households that depend on agriculture and fishing as their main livelihood got only 7.5 percent of their total food from their own production (mainly farming) and only 4.5 percent from wages in kind (mainly fishing).

Gifts and transfers represented the second most important source of food, or around 6 percent of total food expenditures. The share of food from gifts and transfers accounted for almost 8 percent of total consumption for households in the lowest quintile and was significantly higher than for households in the higher quintiles. Households engaged in agriculture relied on gifts and transfers for 8.9 percent of total food expenditures, petty traders for 7–8 percent, and the unemployed for almost 14 percent. Households with income from protected wage labor and self-employment in productive activities—that is, with relatively secure incomes—relied more heavily on purchased food. Gifts and transfers accounted for a significantly higher share of food consumption in indigenous households in Accra than in migrant households.[29] Similarly, female-headed households relied more on transfers for food (9 percent of total food consumption) than households headed by men.

The Kinds of Foods Households Buy

Researchers collected information on more than 160 food items (grouped into 14 food categories) for a seven-day period. Ten groups included unprepared purchased foods and four included prepared foods. Prepared foods are already cooked and ready to eat and are obtained outside the home. This category includes Accra's street foods: snacks, porridges, prepared staple foods, and prepared meals consisting of a staple food item, a soup or sauce, and sometimes a piece of fish, meat, or egg.[30] Cigarettes, alcoholic beverages, and nonalcoholic beverages are not included in this definition of street foods.

Grains, cereals, roots, and tubers dominate the total food consumption basket in Ghana for both urban and rural households. According to the latest GLSS (1991–92), 41.3 percent of the total food budget went toward purchasing these commodities. In Accra, 28 percent of total food outlays went toward purchasing cereals

---

[29] In addition to direct receipts of food, households also receive cash transfers that are used to obtain food. The data on food received as gifts captures the former. Cash transfers that were used to purchase food are captured under "purchases."

[30] Tinker's definition of street foods includes "any minimally processed food sold on the street for immediate consumption" and "purchased food that could be eaten on the spot but that was carried home or to the office" (Tinker 1997, 15).

and roots and tubers. The country's most common staple foods are dough prepared from maize (*banku, kenkey*), millet or sorghum (*tuo zaafi*), and cassava, yams, and plantains (*fufu, konkonte, gari*). In urban centers, wheat bread and fermented porridge are widely consumed as breakfast foods, and rice is becoming more popular.

The mean budget share for cereals and roots and tubers is 23 percent (Table 25). Meat and fish are the next most important commodity group, accounting for 16 percent of total food outlays. Vegetables, fats and oils, and eggs and dairy are also important food items, accounting for more than 18 percent of the average food budget. Street foods account for one-third of total food expenditures, of which more than half goes for prepared meals.

Better-off households have a relatively diversified diet containing foods from animal as well as vegetable sources. Low-income households have a less diversified diet and are more likely to consume large amounts of staple foods. Case studies of very low-income households revealed that staples are the only food these households can afford a good deal of the time. Within the staple foods category, grains and cereals account for a significantly higher share of the food budget in low-income households. However, there are no significant differences in the budget shares for roots and tubers across income groups. Households in the highest expenditure group allocate a significantly higher share of their food budget to foods in the nonstaple category, including fruits and vegetables, meat and fish, and eggs and dairy products, and to nonalcoholic beverages such as tea, coffee, and soft drinks.

Urban consumption patterns are less dominated by staple foods than rural consumption patterns. Urban households allocate more of their food budget to complimentary food groups such as meat and fish, vegetables, fats and oils, and dairy products and eggs (Alderman and Higgins 1992). Differences in incomes between rural and urban households are likely to influence diets, but other factors are also important. Differences in livelihood strategies and time constraints in urban areas, for instance, have increased the consumption of street foods.

Consumption of Street Foods

Urban consumers in Accra purchase a wide variety of foods away from home to meet their needs throughout the day. The majority of these foods are found on the street, including snacks, breakfast foods such as porridge, and lunches, which generally consist of a prepared staple food dish and a soup or stew. Almost all households purchase some prepared food away from home, and a number of households are almost totally dependent on street foods (Figure 5). Among households in the lowest expenditure quintile, 39 percent of the total food budget goes to purchasing snacks and meals away from home (Table 26 and Figure 6). Households in the highest expenditure category spend about 25 percent of their total food budget on street foods.

Street food consumption is related not only to income but also to other factors, including whether women in the household work, the kinds of time constraints that affect principal homemakers, income fluctuations, proximity to markets, and household demographics. The high level of street food purchases may indicate that the

Table 25—Mean share of the food budget spent on different food groups

Category	Number of households	Per capita food expenditures	Grains	Roots/ tubers	Legumes	Vegetables	Fruits	Meat and fish	Eggs and dairy
		(cedis)				(percent)			
Entire sample	559	484,709	14.2	9.0	2.0	7.5	2.1	15.6	5.3
Expenditure group									
1	114	230,763	15.8	10.2	1.7	6.7	1.9	12.3	2.5
2	111	351,167	15.5	9.8	2.1	7.8	1.6	14.1	4.3
3	112	429,163	15.0	8.3	1.9	6.8	2.1	14.2	4.9
4	111	577,082	13.7	8.9	2.1	8.0	2.2	16.8	6.4
5	111	837,077	10.8	7.5	2.2	8.1	2.7	20.7	8.6
Occupational categories[a]									
Agriculture/fishing	13	479,106	15.7	11.0	2.3	8.9	2.0	19.6	4.5
Petty trader	95	485,975	14.6	9.3	2.2	7.4	2.7	14.4	4.6
Street food vendor	47	478,298	14.2	8.9	1.0	6.1	1.4	13.5	4.0
Business	59	557,179	14.0	9.2	1.7	7.9	2.0	18.7	7.3
Skilled labor	149	462,872	14.3	8.6	1.7	7.0	1.9	16.0	4.7
Unskilled labor	69	389,127	16.0	9.5	2.6	7.3	2.1	13.4	4.0
Professional	79	565,135	11.9	8.1	2.6	8.9	2.4	17.6	8.1
Occupation unclassified	7	475,344	14.7	10.4	1.4	10.7	3.0	15.7	4.9
Unemployed	37	474,291	13.8	8.8	2.1	6.9	1.9	13.5	5.7
Migration status of household head									
Indigenous	178	535,913	12.2	6.7	1.8	6.6	1.9	15.7	6.0
Born in Accra—not indigenous	121	473,341	14.6	9.6	2.0	8.4	2.3	16.3	4.6
Migrant	260	454,830	15.4	10.2	2.2	7.7	2.2	15.2	5.2
Sex of head of household									
Male	363		14.3	8.9	2.1	7.6	2.1	16.4	5.6
Female	196		13.9	9.1	1.8	7.3	2.1	14.1	4.8

(continued)

Table 25—Continued

Category	Number of households	Fats and oils	Spices/ condiments	Beverages	Snacks	Prepared porridge	Prepared staples only	Meals
				(percent)				
Entire sample	559	5.4	2.3	4.0	7.7	1.9	3.7	19.4
Expenditure group								
1	114	5.7	2.4	1.9	7.2	2.9	4.7	17.7
2	111	5.4	2.5	3.0	7.6	2.0	4.0	20.4
3	112	5.3	2.1	3.2	7.6	1.8	4.5	22.1
4	111	5.4	2.1	5.9	8.6	1.7	2.6	15.6
5	111	5.2	2.2	6.0	7.7	1.2	2.4	14.7
Occupational categories[a]								
Agriculture/fishing	13	5.5	3.3	1.1	8.0	3.0	1.6	13.7
Petty trader	95	5.2	2.3	3.9	8.5	2.1	3.6	19.4
Street food vendor	47	4.7	1.9	2.2	8.3	2.7	5.7	25.5
Business	59	6.4	2.2	4.3	6.1	1.4	3.0	16.0
Skilled labor	149	5.4	2.3	3.9	7.6	1.8	3.9	20.8
Unskilled labor	69	5.7	2.3	2.9	8.2	2.2	3.7	20.1
Professional	79	5.3	2.2	6.6	7.6	1.2	3.2	14.4
Occupation unclassified	7	5.1	2.2	6.5	8.4	1.9	2.4	12.9
Unemployed	37	4.7	2.2	3.0	7.6	2.6	3.4	24.0
Migration status of household head								
Indigenous	178	5.3	2.0	4.9	8.7	2.0	5.2	20.9
Born in Accra—not indigenous	121	5.5	2.5	4.3	6.9	2.1	3.2	17.8
Migrant	260	5.4	2.4	3.2	7.4	1.8	2.8	19.1
Sex of head of household								
Male	363	5.4	2.3	4.2	7.4	1.8	3.6	18.4
Female	196	5.4	2.2	3.6	8.4	2.2	3.8	21.2

Source: Accra Study Team 1998.
[a] Primary job of household head.

Figure 5—Distribution of the budget share for snacks and prepared foods purchased away from home

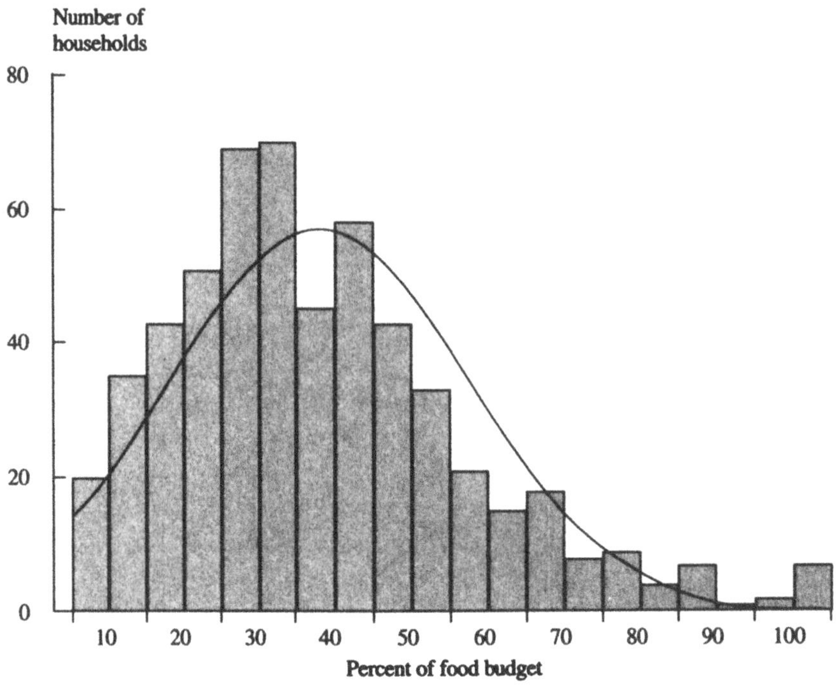

Source: Accra Study Team 1998.

urban poor need to buy food daily because they are short of cash. One seasonally unemployed fisherman commented, "... so when I don't have money to buy food, I just buy *kenkey* and fish." His point is the relative "divisibility" of street foods—even a small amount of money can always buy something from the street, even if the food is not nutritionally adequate.

Urban consumers increasingly rely on prepared foods and snacks in an effort to save the time required to prepare food at home. Street food vendors themselves consume more street foods than any other group, followed by the unemployed and casual labor—occupational groups that have some of the lowest incomes. Indigenous households allocate a significantly higher share of their food budgets to street foods than migrant households. School children also rely on street foods to meet a large share of their daily food requirements. Principal homemakers estimated that of their monthly allocation of money for street foods, 51 percent was spent by or for children. Very young children (4–5 years of age) are often given money for street foods and allowed to buy what they want (Ga Mashie Study Team 1996). This practice made for a special methodological problem for the survey. Principal homemakers often could not answer questions about what even small children in their households had eaten. To circumvent this problem, researchers conducted separate inter-

Table 26—Mean share of food budget allocated to street foods and meals away from home

Category	Number of households	Street foods and meals away from home
Entire sample	559	32.7
Expenditure group		
1	114	39.1
2	111	33.9
3	112	36.1
4	111	25.9
5	111	25.5
Occupational categories[a]		
Agriculture/fishing	13	26.3
Petty trader	95	33.5
Street food vendor	47	42.2
Business	59	26.4
Skilled labor	149	34.1
Unskilled labor	69	34.2
Professional	79	26.3
Occupation unclassified	7	25.5
Unemployed	37	37.5
Migration status of household head		
Indigenous	178	36.9
Born in Accra—not indigenous	121	30.0
Migrant	260	31.1
Sex of head of household		
Male	363	31.1
Female	196	35.7

Source: Accra Study Team 1998.
[a] Primary job of household head.

views with any household member who had consumed street foods in the last 30 days. While extremely time-consuming, this approach yielded better consumption estimates and probably more accurate estimates of household expenditures on food—especially of spending on street foods.

Food Availability

Studies have shown that urban diets are strongly influenced by prices and incomes, but they are also influenced by lifestyles, social relationships, marriage patterns, family structures, the availability of packaged and processed foods, advertising, and the media (Austin et al. 1976; Chaudhri and Timmer 1986; Drakakis-Smith 1991; von Braun et al. 1993; Atkinson 1995; Boughton and Reardon 1997; Randolph 1997; Tinker 1997). Processed and packaged foods are more widely available in urban than in rural areas, in part because food manufacturing sectors are based nearby. Urban markets are also likely to carry imported food items.

Figure 6—Share of food expenditures spent on street foods and meals away from home, by expenditure group

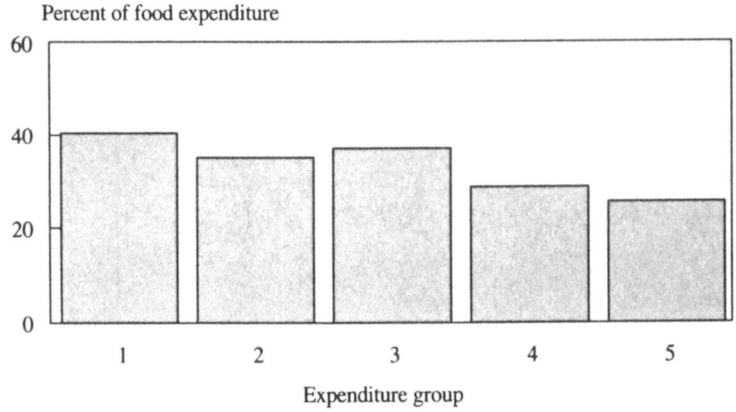

Source: Accra Study Team 1998.
Notes: Group 1 is the lowest expenditure group; group 5 the highest.

However, how the nutritional value of urban diets is affected by these factors is not well understood. Do shifts in consumption toward more expensive staple foods compromise the diet? How does increased consumption of street food contribute to calorie intake? This section addresses these questions by presenting evidence on the availability of calories at the household level and then analyzing the major sources of calories.

Caloric Intake

The mean availability of calories at the household level for the entire sample is approximately 2,640 kilocalories per adult equivalent units per day (kcal/aeu/day) (Table 27). This figure falls well within the range of previous studies of food availability in Ghana (Alderman and Higgins 1992; Brown and Kerr 1997; Asenso-Okyere, Asante, and Nubé 1997). The number of available calories increases with income, with mean availability ranging from 1,785 kcal/aeu/day for the lowest expenditure group to 3,309 kcal/aeu/day for the highest expenditure quintile. The mean price per calorie was 749 per 1,000 kcal. The mean cost per 1,000 calories for the lowest income group was roughly 580. To get the recommended number of calories, then, individuals in this quintile would have to spend roughly ₵1,680 per aeu/day.[31] The average household contained 3.4 aeu and so would have to spend around ₵5,700 per day in order to provide minimum calories. This figure is well above the daily *total* household expenditure for some 16 percent of the sample. In

[31] The recommended number is 2,900 kcal/aeu/day.

Table 27—Mean daily calorie availability

Category	Number of households	Calories per AEU[a]	Price per 1,000 calories
Expenditure group			
1	111	1,785.8	581.0
2	111	2,420.2	647.0
3	112	2,622.7	695.0
4	111	3,024.7	805.7
5	111	3,309.1	1,004.4
Occupational categories[b]			
Agriculture/fishing	13	2,711.4	658.4
Petty trader	99	2,771.3	729.4
Street food vendor	47	2,846.4	720.7
Business	59	2,659.0	797.3
Skilled labor	149	2,551.5	730.9
Unskilled labor	69	2,389.4	657.0
Professional	78	2,586.3	886.9
Unclassified	7	2,600.1	661.8
Unemployed	37	2,812.7	717.9
Migration status of household head			
Indigenous	178	2,672.3	823.2
Born in Accra—not indigenous	121	2,755.4	717.5
Migrant	259	2,549.2	706.4
Sex of household head			
Male	362	2,552.9	749.2
Female	196	2,781.5	740.3
Total	559	2,633.2	746.0

Source: Study Team 1998.
Note: Unadjusted for guests.
[a] Adult equivalent unit.
[b] Primary job of head of household.

terms of calories, then, some low-income groups in Accra simply do not earn enough to afford an adequate diet.

The calorie shares do not correspond to the budget shares presented in Table 26, because foods that are relatively expensive sources of calories have higher budget shares than calorie shares (Alderman and Higgins 1992) (Table 28). Roots and tubers, grains and cereals, and fats and oils are relatively cheap sources of foods, while meat and fish, eggs and dairy, and vegetables are more expensive. For instance, the mean budget share for oil was 5.4 percent. Yet fats and oils make up almost 12 percent of total household calorie availability. Similarly, meats and fish account for 14 percent of total food expenditures but contribute only 6 percent to total household calories. Roots and tubers are a cheaper source of staple foods, yet for the sample as a whole the mean calorie share for grains and cereals is higher than the share for roots and tubers.

Table 28—Mean percent of total calories available from different food groups

Category	N	Grains	Tubers	Legumes	Vegetables	Fruits	Meat and fish	Eggs and dairy
Entire sample	559	24.5	20.8	4.1	1.3	1.7	6.1	1.9
Expenditure group								
1	111	24.6	22.8	3.0	1.1	1.2	4.5	0.7
2	111	27.2	20.6	3.3	1.4	1.1	5.9	1.4
3	112	25.1	19.3	3.9	1.2	1.5	5.2	1.8
4	111	25.0	20.4	4.3	1.4	1.9	6.4	2.3
5	111	20.6	20.6	5.6	1.5	2.7	8.7	3.2
Occupational categories[a]								
Agriculture/fishing	13	26.6	23.0	6.6	1.8	1.6	7.9	1.3
Petty trader	99	23.5	22.1	4.2	1.3	2.1	5.1	1.9
Street food vendor	47	23.3	18.5	1.8	1.1	1.1	4.7	1.5
Business	59	25.6	22.7	3.9	1.2	1.6	6.1	2.4
Skilled labor	149	24.7	19.9	3.3	1.3	1.4	6.7	1.8
Unskilled labor	69	27.6	20.6	4.7	1.4	1.7	5.8	1.5
Professional	78	22.8	21.3	5.5	1.4	2.1	7.5	2.6
Occupation unclassified	7	26.4	23.0	2.5	1.8	2.2	7.9	0.9
Unemployed	37	22.4	18.3	4.9	1.1	1.6	5.1	1.9
Migration status of household head								
Indigenou	178	21.9	17.3	3.7	1.2	1.7	5.9	2.5
Born in Accra—not indigenous	121	25.7	22.3	3.5	1.4	1.7	6.7	1.6
Migrant	259	25.7	22.4	4.6	1.3	1.7	5.9	1.7
Sex of household head								
Male	362	24.9	21.1	4.4	1.3	1.7	6.7	1.9
Female	196	23.6	20.1	3.4	1.3	1.7	5.1	1.8

(continued)

Table 28—Continued

Category	Number of household	Fats and oils	Spices/ condiments	Beverages	Snacks	Prepared porridge	Prepared staples only	Meals
Entire sample	559	12.2	0.1	0.3	5.3	0.8	4.0	16.9
Expenditure group								
1	111	10.5	0.1	0.1	4.4	1.2	4.7	21.2
2	111	11.4	0.1	0.1	4.8	0.9	4.5	17.4
3	112	11.6	0.1	0.2	5.0	0.7	4.4	19.9
4	111	13.4	0.1	0.5	6.1	0.7	3.3	14.1
5	111	13.9	0.1	0.6	6.1	0.5	3.4	12.4
Occupational categories[a]								
Agriculture/fishing	13	10.6	0.1	0.0	5.9	1.5	1.6	11.4
Petty trader	99	11.6	0.1	0.2	5.7	0.9	3.9	17.4
Street food vendor	47	11.0	0.1	0.1	5.5	0.8	6.2	24.2
Business	59	14.8	0.1	0.2	4.4	0.5	3.8	12.4
Skilled labor	149	12.2	0.1	0.3	5.0	0.8	4.9	17.4
Unskilled labor	69	11.4	0.1	0.2	5.2	0.9	2.9	15.9
Professional	78	13.2	0.1	0.6	5.6	0.6	2.9	13.8
Occupation unclassified	7	10.8	0.1	0.2	6.7	0.2	4.0	13.0
Unemployed	37	10.7	0.1	0.3	5.2	0.9	4.0	23.4
Migration status of household head								
Indigenous	178	12.8	0.1	0.4	6.2	0.9	5.9	19.4
Born in Accra—not indigenous	121	11.9	0.1	0.3	4.9	0.9	2.9	16.0
Migrant	259	11.8	0.1	0.2	4.8	0.7	3.3	15.7
Sex of household head								
Male	362	12.1	9.2	0.3	5.2	0.8	3.9	15.4
Female	196	12.2	6.8	0.2	5.4	0.8	4.2	19.8

Source: Accra Study Team 1998.
[a]Primary job of household head.

Although calorie availability did not differ significantly across occupational status or migration status of head of household, costs differed markedly across these categories. There were no significant differences in costs between male- and female-headed households, yet mean calorie availability was significantly higher for households headed by women. In general, the types of food consumed by households at various income levels explain these differences. Poorer households—including many headed by women—get more of their calories from starchy staples than wealthier households. As household income increases, the average diet becomes more diversified. Households with higher incomes get fewer of their total calories from staples such as grains and cereals and more from legumes, vegetables, fruits, meat and fish, dairy products, fats and oils, beverages, and snack foods.

As has been noted, urban residents tend to rely heavily on street foods and meals purchased away from home. A large share of total calories comes from these prepared foods. The mean calorie share for street foods or prepared meals purchased away from home was 27 percent for the entire sample (Table 29). The total amount of calories obtained from street and other prepared foods was significantly higher

Table 29—Mean percent of total calories available from street foods and meals away from home

Category	Number of households	Percent
Expenditure group		
1	111	31.4
2	111	27.5
3	112	30.0
4	111	24.3
5	111	22.5
Occupational categories[a]		
Agriculture/fishing	13	20.4
Petty trader	99	28.0
Street food vendor	47	36.7
Business	59	21.2
Skilled labor	149	28.2
Unskilled labor	69	24.9
Professional	78	22.9
Unclassified	7	23.9
Unemployed	37	33.5
Migration status of household head		
Indigenous	178	32.5
Born in Accra—not indigenous	121	24.8
Migrant	259	24.5
Sex of household head		
Male	362	25.4
Female	196	30.3
Total	559	27.1

Source: Accra Study Team 1998.
[a] Primary job of household head.

for households in the lowest income group, accounting for just over 30 percent of total calorie availability. Indigenous households obtained significantly more of their calories from prepared foods than migrant households, and female-headed households had higher calorie shares from these foods than male-headed households. Calories from prepared meals accounted for almost 62 percent of all calories purchased away from home.

Food Contamination

Qualitative investigations suggest a strong link between reliance on street foods and the prevalence of gastrointestinal infections, presumably because street foods are easily contaminated. This connection manifested itself in complaints of diarrhea or "upset stomach," conditions that were often blamed on poorly cooked food or the sanitary conditions under which the food was prepared or sold (Ga Mashie Study Team 1996). However, case study informants repeatedly mentioned that they knew which street food sellers were careful in preparing their foods and practiced acceptable levels of cleanliness. One mother noted, "Don't you see those women selling food by the big drain [an open sewer]? Flies land on their food, and if we eat it, we get sick." Street food vendors are aware of this problem as well. One noted, "If you do not cook [the food] well, everyone will boycott you, because what you are selling is being sold by dozens of people in the same vicinity. . . . "

Levels of contamination in street foods may indeed be high (FAO 1996). Akpedonu (1996) reports that in general, snack foods purchased on the streets of Accra are safe from bacterial contamination. But she notes that prepared meals, and especially uncooked vegetables (in salad condiments served with prepared meals, for example), have high levels of contamination. This study did not test the relationship between street food consumption and individual health outcomes. However, other studies on food contamination in Accra (Mensah et al. 1995) note that levels of contamination in foods prepared at home may also be high. Thus street foods may not be the only cause of bacterial gastrointestinal infections.

Coping with Limited Food

As pointed out in Chapter 4, individuals and households have a variety of strategies for coping with financial shortfalls. Case studies noted a number of strategies households employed at times when there was not enough money to buy food for all household members. In generic terms, these include dietary changes such as buying cheaper and less-preferred foods (maize and cassava, for instance), temporary measures to increase the amount of food available or reduce the number of people who have to be fed, and rationing or somehow "managing" the shortfall in available food. Nine commonly practiced strategies were identified through focus groups and case studies and included in the survey (Table 30).

The data in Table 30 show considerable differences in the frequency with which households employ the various coping strategies. Over three-fourths of the households

Table 30—Coping strategies related to food consumption: Frequencies and proportions

Strategy	Relative frequency in past month						
	Every day	3–6 times/ week	1–2 times/ week	<1 time/ week	Never	Mean score[a] (S.D.)	Number
1. Relying on less preferred and less expensive food	9 (1.6%)	94 (16.8%)	166 (29.7%)	160 (28.6%)	127 (22.7%)	1.46 (1.67)	556
2. Borrowing food, or money to purchase food	1 (0.2%)	12 (2.1%)	33 (5.9%)	59 (10.6%)	453 (81.0%)	0.25 (0.78)	558
3. Purchasing food on credit	1 (0.2%)	45 (8.1%)	50 (9.3%	63 (11.3%)	427 (76.4%)	0.33 (0.89)	557
4. Relying on assistance from a friend or relative outside the household	24 (4.3%)	45 (8.1%)	52 (9.3%)	80 (14.3%)	357 (63.9%)	0.87 (1.79)	557
5. Rationing by limiting portion size at mealtimes	4 (0.%)	45 (8.1%)	117 (20.9%)	145 (25.9%)	247 (44.2%)	0.85 (1.33)	558
6. Rationing by purchasing street foods with the available cash	10 (1.8%)	97 (17.4%)	117 (20.9%)	138 (24.7%)	195 (34.9%)	1.34 (1.76)	557
7. Rationing by limiting intake of adults so children get enough to eat	9 (1.6%)	67 (12.0%)	138 (24.7%)	154 (27.2%)	192 (34.3%)	1.16 (1.58)	558
8. Rationing by reducing the number of meals per day	8 (1.4%)	27 (4.8%)	60 (10.7%)	105 (18.8%)	358 (64.0%)	0.57 (1.28)	558
9. Skipping whole days without eating	. . .	1 (0.2%)	3 (0.6%)	5 (1.2%)	546 (97.7%)	0.02 0.22	557

Source: Accra Study Team 1998.

Note: Interpretation of mean scores: The higher the mean score, the more frequently the study population relies on this coping strategy. The numbers in parentheses are the percent of respondents who use this coping strategy. Sample includes both households and individuals.

[a] Raw score: Every day = 7; 3–6 times/week = 4.5; 1–2 times/week = 1.5; Less than 1 time/week = 0.5; Never = 0.

in the sample conserve on expenses by eating cheaper, less-preferred food. Rationing money for the purchase of street food is the second-most common coping strategy—a finding consistent with Norton et al. (1995).[32] Households that reported relying heavily on street foods as a coping strategy shared several characteristics. They also reported a significantly higher share of prepared food in total consumption than other households, a significantly lower level of food expenditures per capita, and a significantly higher share of expenditure on food overall.

Among this group of households, there was a strong positive linear relationship between the frequency with which they used this coping strategy and the share of prepared food in the diet. This share reached almost 60 percent of food expenditures in the group that reported using street foods as a coping strategy most frequently. And there was a strong negative linear relationship between the frequency of the coping strategy and total expenditure on food. Total mean food expenditures in the group that reported using the coping strategy less than once a week were ₵523,000 per capita. But in the group that reported using this coping strategy every day, expenditures were only ₵31,000 per capita. These results verify that relying on street foods and rationing money to buy them are important strategies in Accra for households without enough money to purchase food. One unemployed man put it this way: "The little we have just goes for *kenkey* and fish, or sometimes just *kenkey* and pepper. We just try to fill our stomachs—we have no alternative. . . . "

Mothers and primary homemakers practiced the third most common coping strategy: limiting their food intake in order to ensure that children had enough to eat. Skipping meals for an entire day, clearly the most drastic of any of the strategies mentioned, was the option practiced least frequently. In the qualitative community and household case studies, respondents often spoke of having to borrow food or money as a source of shame, and undoubtedly for that reason this strategy is the second to last in popularity. Nevertheless, the evidence in Chapter 4 suggests that borrowing money is common and that the money is often spent on food. The difference, as expressed in follow-up focus groups, is that borrowing money is not considered shameful, but having to borrow food is.[33] There are also strong cultural differences in attitudes toward borrowing.[34]

Household Food Security

One important objective of the study was to estimate as accurately as possible the proportion of households in Accra that are not able to maintain food security. Household

---

[32] It should be reiterated, however, that consuming street foods does not always indicate a shortfall in food or cash at the household level. Total consumption levels of street food are much higher than reported here.

[33] For this reason, someone lending money may not know what it was used for or may be reluctant to say in order not to insult a close friend or relative.

[34] The coping strategies described here have also been compiled into an index according to frequency and severity that can be used as an alternative indicator of household food security. See Maxwell et al. (1999).

food security is defined as access by all people at all times to enough food to ensure an active, healthy life.[35] Since only a single round of data was collected, the study does not shed light on certain questions. It was not able to document fluctuations in urban food consumption throughout the year or determine whether households' experience chronic or transitory food insecurity. Qualitative results indicate that some predictable seasonal variations in household food availability are tied to certain livelihoods—notably fishing and farming, both of which are becoming less and less common (Ga Mashie Study Team 1996; Ngleshie Amanfro Study Team 1996). However, the same results indicate that the seasonal fluctuations in food consumption in other households depends on unpredictable factors such as illness or injury or loss of a job or income earner—in other words, livelihood-related factors, not seasonal changes.

Food prices vary significantly with the season and so may affect the amount of food households are able to purchase. Alderman and Shively (1996) note a difference of 50 percent in the real price of maize in urban markets between June (the preharvest season) and September (the postharvest season). Prices for other food commodities follow this trend, although the magnitude of the difference varies. The survey took place about halfway between the postharvest and preharvest periods, when food prices were roughly average in real terms.

There is no single indicator that best measures household food security, so several are used here. One common indicator is calorie adequacy (Payne 1990; Habicht and Pelletier 1990; Maxwell and Frankenberger 1992; Haddad, Kennedy, and Sullivan 1994; S. Maxwell 1996; Chung et al. 1997). This measure captures food sufficiency in terms of quantity but does not address the quality of the diet or issues of vulnerability or sustainable access. The traditional approach to measuring household food security using dietary intakes has been to select an optimal caloric intake based on a recommended daily allowance (RDA) for the equivalent of a moderately active adult and compare it to observed household caloric intake per adult equivalent.

In order to identify households that are experiencing food insecurity, researchers used a cutoff point for caloric intake. This technique presents two problems. The first is how to determine the correct cutoff point in the absence of full information for estimating the energy requirements of the sample.[36] The second, more general

---

[35] A full definition of food security includes the related concepts of access, sufficiency, vulnerability, and sustainability put forth in Maxwell and Frankenberger (1992).

[36] It is not possible to quantify energy requirements, because the study did not collect data on weights and time allocation or measure activity levels for all household members. The estimated energy requirement used for this study was derived from the 1981 Estimated Average Requirements for the United Kingdom, Department of Health and Social Security, as presented in Gibson (1990). These figures were chosen for two reasons. First, the recommendations are broken down for 30 different combinations of age, sex, activity level, and physiological status, providing a level of detail not seen in other similar tabulations. Second, the average required intake for adult women (2,150 kilocalories) closely matched the estimated requirement for Accra women in the sample based on their age, weight, and a physical activity level factor of 1.64. Other tabulations suggested lower intakes for this population group. Since the U.K. figures did not include recommendations for infants (<1 year), these were taken from *Energy and Protein Requirements* (IDECG 1994, S33). The recommended daily allowance used for this study is 2,900 kcal/aeu/day.

issue is whether or not applying certain calorie requirements makes sense, given the fluctuations in household and individual dietary requirements and individuals' ability to adjust to inadequate energy intakes (Beaton 1983; Dugdale and Payne 1987; Edmundson and Sukhatme 1990). Given these caveats, calorie adequacy can be evaluated using several cutoffs. The first cutoff is 80 percent of the RDA (2,320 kcal/aeu/day). The second is 2,200 kcal/aeu/day, a number that has been used in previous studies to measure calorie adequacy in Ghana and elsewhere (Kennedy et al. 1994; Haddad 1993; Brown and Kerr 1997). A somewhat more complex method of categorizing food insecurity builds on the model proposed by Jonsson and Toole (1991). This model considers both calorie adequacy and the proportion of the total household budget devoted to food.

Household Calorie (Energy) Adequacy

Based on the recommendation of 2,900 kcal/aeu/day, the overall adequacy for the sample is 91 percent. The mean household calorie availability in the two highest expenditure groups is over 100 percent of required intake (Table 31). But this figure

Table 31—Mean percentage of energy adequacy per adult equivalent unit

Category	Number of households	Percent
Expenditure group		
1	111	62.0
2	111	83.0
3	112	90.0
4	111	104.0
5	111	114.0
Occupational categories[a]		
Agriculture/fishing	13	93.0
Petty trader	99	96.0
Street food vendor	47	98.0
Business	59	92.0
Skilled labor	149	88.0
Unskilled labor	69	82.0
Professional	78	89.0
Unclassified	7	90.0
Unemployed	37	97.0
Migration status of household head		
Indigenous	178	92.0
Born in Accra—not indigenous	121	95.0
Migrant	259	88.0
Sex of household head		
Male	362	88.0
Female	196	96.0
Total	559	91.0

Source: Accra Study Team 1998.
[a] Primary job of household head.

Table 32—Mean percentage of energy-deficient households

Category	Number of households	Below 80% of calorie requirement	Below 2,200 kcal/aeu/day
Expenditure group			
1	111	80.0	78.0
2	111	54.0	45.0
3	112	36.0	34.0
4	111	23.0	21.0
5	111	10.0	10.0
Occupational categories[a]			
Agriculture/fishing	13	31.0	31.0
Petty trader	99	34.0	31.0
Street food vendor	47	34.0	32.0
Business	59	46.0	41.0
Skilled labor	149	40.0	38.0
Unskilled labor	69	54.0	51.0
Professional	78	45.0	40.0
Unclassified	7	43.0	43.0
Unemployed	37	27.0	27.0
Migration status of household head			
Indigenous	178	40.0	38.0
Born in Accra, indigenous	121	35.0	33.0
Migrant	259	43.0	39.0
Sex of household head			
Male	362	44.0	40.0
Female	196	34.0	32.0
Total	559	40.0	37.0

Source: Accra Study Team 1998.
[a] Primary job of household head.

is roughly 60 percent of required intake for households in the lowest expenditure quintile. There are no significant differences in the mean energy adequacy across occupation or migration status. Female-headed households, which have significantly higher calorie availability (at the same price per 1,000 calories), also have significantly higher mean calorie adequacy.

There is a strong relationship between expenditures and calorie adequacy. In the group with the lowest expenditures, 80 percent of the households fall below 80 percent of the calorie requirement and 78 percent fall below 2,200 kcal/aeu/day (Table 32). In the group with the highest income, only 10 percent of the households do not meet the calorie requirement.

The relationship between calorie adequacy and expenditure becomes less clear when occupation, migration, and sex of the household head are taken into account. The occupational groups associated with relatively high mean incomes in Chapter 4 do not necessarily have the fewest households below the cutoff for calorie adequacy. Households whose heads are employed as skilled or unskilled laborers, engaged in professional services, or self-employed in business are more likely to fall below both cutoffs. Meanwhile, the percentage of calorie-deficient households is lowest for occupational groups such as agriculture and fishing, street food vending, and petty trading. The agriculture and fishing group is very small, as is the group of households with unemployed heads, but these two groups had the smallest percentage of households classified as "food insecure" using the calorie cutoffs. Among female-headed households, which have lower mean incomes than male-headed households, the percentage of households falling below either cutoff was significantly lower. A number of factors may explain these trends.

First, the mean income levels may be masking the number of poor households found within occupational groups. For instance, while the mean income for professionals may be higher than for other categories, this group still contains vulnerable households without enough income to obtain sufficient food for all household members. Second, energy requirements should vary according to the level of physical activity required for each job. Business and professional occupations may be rather sedentary jobs that require less energy (and therefore fewer calories) than agricultural work or skilled and unskilled labor. Even within occupational categories, activity levels—and thus calorie requirements—may vary. Petty trading and street food vending, for example, may be more or less physically demanding, depending on whether the trader or vendor is itinerant or stationed at a permanent stall.

Third, there is a fairly clear difference in spending priorities between male- and female-headed households. Female-headed households spend an average of 60 percent of their total resources on food, whereas male-headed households spend just over 50 percent of their resources on food. Female-headed households buy slightly cheaper calories as well, and thus a lower proportion of female-headed households are calorie deficient. Female-headed households also tend to fall into the occupational groups that have the lowest proportions of households below the cutoff points for calorie adequacy—specifically street food vendors and petty traders. Male-headed households are much more likely to be in occupational groups such as casual or unskilled labor. Finally, type and source of income may play an important role in allowing female-headed households to secure adequate calories. These households receive the largest share of total income from cash and in-kind transfers of any household group.

Calorie Adequacy and Budget Shares

Calorie availability was also cross-classified with food shares. A cutoff of 80 percent of the calorie requirement was combined with a food share greater than 60 percent of total expenditure for the top figure or 50 percent for the lower figure in Table 33.[37] Classifying the data in this way adds a dimension of vulnerability to an essentially cross-sectional indicator. Households in group 1 are clearly food secure—

[37] The figure 2,320 is 80 percent of 2,900 kcal, the recommended requirement for an adult of average size in Ghana; 60 percent is the mean food expenditure for the lowest two expenditure quintiles in the sample.

Table 33—Food security: Caloric adequacy and food shares

	Share of expenditure on food	
	Low **a:(<60% of budget share)** **b:(<50% of budget share)**	**High** **a:(>60% of budget share)** **b:(>50% of budget share)**
Caloric availability per adult equivalent unit	1. Food Secure	2. Vulnerable
Adequate (>80% of requirement)	a:182 (32.8%) b:115 (20.6%)	a:148 (26.7%) b:219 (39.2%)
Inadequate (<80% of requirement)	3. Questionable: (Can improve consumption, or measurement error) a:149 (26.8%) b:93 (16.6%)	4. Food insecure a:76 (13.7%) b:132 (23.6%)

Source: Adapted from Jonsson and Toole 1991.

Note: Number and percentages in each group refer to numbers of households and proportion of the total sample.

an indication of relative security from shocks. Their food consumption is adequate and they spend a relatively small proportion of the budget on food. Households in group 4 are clearly food insecure. Their consumption is inadequate, and they spend a large share of their budget on food. Group 2 might be labeled vulnerable, with current consumption adequate but a high proportion of the budget allocated to food. A relatively small shock could lower consumption for this group. Group 3 has low consumption but also low food shares and is thus more difficult to explain. The findings could be a measurement error—that is, households could have underreported either food consumption or over reported nonfood expenditures. The recall period could simply have been unrepresentative, with unusually high nonfood expenditures. The findings could also be explained in terms of a deliberate trade-off between food consumption and other necessities, including savings, investment or remittances, and basic consumption needs (de Waal 1989).

In fact, all of these factors help to explain why over a quarter of the sampled households have low food consumption and devote a relatively low share of the household budget to food. Lowering the food shares cutoff to 50 percent moves an additional 56 households out of that category and into the "food insecure" category (Table 33). But the cutoff for food shares is then well below the sample mean of 54 percent, and 93 households (17 percent of the sample) still remain in the "questionable" category. Of the 93 households remaining in this category after the cutoff for food shares is lowered to 50 percent, 39 households were "net remitters" sending money to other households. Most of these households (virtually all of which

Table 34—Sociodemographic groups by food security categories

Category	Food secure	Vulnerable	Questionable	Food insecure	Total
1	0	22	20	69	111
	(0.0)	(19.8)	(18.0)	(62.2)	(100)
2	2	49	19	31	111
	(1.8)	(44.1)	(17.1)	(36.9)	(100)
3	12	60	24	16	112
	(10.7)	(53.6)	(21.4)	(14.3)	(100)
4	29	57	19	6	111
	(26.1)	(51.4)	(17.1)	(5.4)	(100)
5	69	31	11	0	111
	(62.2)	(27.9)	(9.1)	(0.0)	(100)
Occupation of head					
Agriculture/fishing	1	8	3	1	13
	(7.7)	(61.5)	(23.1)	(7.7)	(100)
Petty trading	13	52	15	19	99
	(13.1)	(52.5)	(15.2)	(19.2)	(100)
Street food vending	2	29	1	15	47
	(4.3)	(61.7)	(2.1)	(31.9)	(100)
Business	21	11	14	13	59
	(35.6)	(18.6)	(23.7)	(22.0)	(100)
Skilled labor	35	55	29	30	149
	(23.5)	(36.9)	(19.5)	(20.1)	(100)
Unskilled labor	7	25	10	27	69
	(10.1)	(36.2)	(14.5)	(39.1)	(100)
Professional	27	17	20	15	79
	(34.2)	(21.5)	(25.3)	(19.0)	(100)
Unclassified	2	2	0	3	7
	(28.6)	(28.6)	(0.0)	(42.9)	(100)
Unemployed	7	20	1	9	37
	(18.9)	(54.1)	(2.7)	(24.3)	(100)
Migration status of household head					
Indigenous	35	72	29	42	178
	(19.7)	(40.4)	(16.3)	(23.6)	(100)
Not indigenous—born in Accra	28	51	14	28	121
	(23.1)	(42.1)	(11.6)	(23.1)	(100)
Migrant	52	96	50	62	260
	(20.0)	(36.9)	(19.2)	(23.8)	(100)
Headship					
Male	88	117	73	85	363
	(24.2)	(32.2)	(20.1)	(23.4)	(100)
Female	27	102	20	47	196
	(13.8)	(52.0)	(10.2)	(24.0)	(100)
Total	115	219	93	132	559
	(20.6)	(39.2)	(16.6)	(23.6)	(100)

Source: Accra Study Team 1998.
Note: Numbers in parentheses are percentages of respondents.

were migrant) were not receiving any remittances themselves. For this group of households, a trade-off existed between their own consumption and the need to provide money to other households (usually close relatives). Of the remaining households, some were clearly underestimating consumption—the larger the household, the greater the error in the estimate. Others were clearly food insecure but had had unusually large nonfood expenditures during the recall period that made food expenditure appear low when reported as a budget share. Categorizing the households in this group with regard to their food security status is thus very difficult.

Table 34 uses the four categories described above but gives a somewhat different picture of household food security. The expenditure quintile groups continue to tell a relatively predictable story: none of the households in the lowest quintile falls into the "food secure" group, and none in the highest quintile falls into the "food insecure" group. Nearly two-thirds of households in the lowest quintile are "food insecure," and exactly the same proportion of the highest quintile are in the "food secure" group. By occupational category, unskilled labor and street food vendors have the highest proportion in the "food insecure" group. Agriculture, petty trading, and street food vending have the highest proportion in the "vulnerable" group—a rather different picture than the one based solely on calorie availability (which depicted relatively lower proportions falling below the cutoff).

A high proportion of female-headed households have adequate calorie availability levels but are more vulnerable to shocks because they spend a higher proportion of their disposable income to acquire the calories. In the "food insecure" category, there is scarcely any difference between male- and female-headed households or indigenous and migrant groups. Twice as many male-headed households fall into the "questionable" category. A higher proportion of migrants than of indigenous households also falls into this category.

In terms of calorie availability alone, roughly 40 percent of households in the sample can be categorized as food insecure. When the measure of food insecurity includes both calorie availability and the food share of the total budget, some 24 percent are classified as food insecure and about 40 percent as vulnerable. Female-headed households, street food vendors, and petty traders—groups that overlap considerably—are the most vulnerable. These are the same groups that were identified in the previous chapter as being most vulnerable to income shortfalls. (Chapter 10 further analyzes the coping strategies of the various food security groups derived here and discusses the relationship between food security and health and nutritional status).

CHAPTER 6

Nutrition and Health of Women and Children

Previous chapters have shown how Accra's residents earn their livelihoods and described the ways households use their income and other resources to obtain food and meet their basic needs. This chapter presents descriptive information about the health and nutritional status of women and children in Accra. In examining the links between nutrition and health outcomes, it takes into account factors in women's lives that may affect the health of their children.

Nutritional Status of Children

The study collected survey data on the nutritional status of preschool children in the households that made up the sample (Tables 35 and 36).[38] One child from each household—the index child—was studied in depth. The data on childhood malnutrition are presented using the three common anthropometric indicators: height for age, weight for age, and weight for height.[39]

The mean height-for-age Z-scores and weight-for-age Z-scores for all three groups of children are in the range of –0.9 to –1.0. The mean weight-for-height Z-scores are clustered around –0.5 (Table 35). Stunting is more prevalent than wast-

[38] These data were analyzed for three subgroups:

1. Children 3 to 36 months of age, for which the sample is statistically representative of Greater Accra (n = 561);
2. Index children, who, by definition, were between 0 and 36 months of age at the time of the survey but were in practice 0 to 39 months (the maximum age was 38.37 months) (n = 556); and
3. Children 0 to 59 months of age (for which the sample is not statistically representative of Greater Accra) (n = 724).

Unless otherwise indicated, results in this section are presented and discussed for the first subgroup of children (3–36 months old). Of the 559 households in the sample, anthropometric data were missing for three index children, lowering the total number of households represented to 556.

[39] Z-scores were derived using the reference standards developed by the U.S. Center for Disease Control (CDC), The National Center for Health Statistics (CNHS), and the World Health Organization (WHO 1979). Standard cutoff points and definitions are used for malnutrition. Stunting is defined as height-for-age Z-scores below –2.00, underweight as weight-for-age Z-scores below –2.00, and wasting as weight-for-height Z-scores below –2.00.

Table 35—Mean anthropometric measurements of children in Accra, 1997

Age group	Number	Height-for-age Z-score	Weight-for-age Z-score	Weight-for-height Z-score
Children 3–36 months	561	–0.94	–1.05	–0.57
		(1.18)	(1.06)	(0.93)
Index children (0–39 months)	556	–0.87	–0.94	–0.50
		(1.16)	(1.09)	(0.95)
Children under 60 months	724	–0.93	–0.97	–0.48
		(1.19)	(1.08)	(0.93)

Source: Accra Study Team 1998.
Note: Standard deviations are in parentheses.

ing (17.6 percent versus 5.3 percent), a common finding in Sub-Saharan Africa (Victora 1992; Sommerfelt and Stewart 1994).[40]

Height-for-age and weight-for-age Z-scores improve linearly as household expenditures increase (Table 37). Differences in weight-for-height are neither consistent nor statistically significant. Occupational categories are also associated with differences in both height for age and weight for age, but not in weight for height. The lowest nutritional status is found among children from households in which the head's main occupation is street food vending, agriculture or fishing, or unskilled labor. As expected, children who live in households with heads engaged in the pro-

Table 36—Prevalence of malnutrition among children in Accra, 1997

		Stunted (height-for-age Z-score < –2)		Underweight (weight-for-age Z-score < –2)		Wasted (weight-for-height Z-score < –2)	
Age group	Number	Percent[a]	CI	Percent[a]	CI	Percent[a]	CI
Children 3–36 months	561	17.6	[14.6–21.1][b] [14.2–21.7][c]	15.7	[12.8–19.0][b]	5.3	[3.7–7.6][b] [3.5–8.1][c]
Index children (0–39 months)	556	15.6	[12.8–19.0][b] [12.4–19.5][c]	13.3	[10.6–16.5][b]	4.5	[3.0–6.5][b] [2.8–7.1][c]
Children less than 60 months	724	17.3	[14.6–20.3][b] [14.2–20.7][c]	13.4	[11.0–16.1][b]	4.4	[3.1–6.3][b] [2.9–6.6][c]

Source: Accra Study Team 1998.
[a] 95 percent confidence interval (CI).
[b] Uncorrected confidence interval.
[c] Confidence interval corrected for design effect.

[40] The weight-for-age Z-scores and the data on prevalence of underweight children are of limited value because they do not differentiate between stunting and wasting, which have a very different etiology. In the case of Accra, weight-for-age Z-scores happen to reflect height-for-age Z-scores quite accurately because both wasting and overweight (low and high weight for height, respectively) are uncommon among young children. In this case, weight-for-height Z-scores can be used as a proxy for stunting when height-length data are not available.

Table 37—Nutritional status of children by household characteristics, 1997

Household characteristics	Number	Height-for-age Z-score	Weight-for-age Z-score	Weight-for-height Z-score
Entire sample	557	–0.87	–0.94	–0.49
Expenditure group				
1	110	–1.05	–1.19	–0.67
2	110	–0.94	–0.92	–0.43
3	112	–0.91	–0.93	–0.42
4	111	–0.78	–0.90	–0.52
5	111	–0.65	–0.78	–0.43
Occupational category of household head				
Agriculture/fishing	13	–1.16	–0.83	–0.27
Petty trader	99	–0.96	–0.94	–0.41
Street food vendor	47	–1.23	–1.32	–0.72
Business	59	–0.82	–0.89	–0.48
Skilled labor	149	–0.81	–0.88	–0.45
Unskilled labor	70	–1.11	–1.22	–0.67
Professional	78	–0.45	–0.72	–0.50
Occupation unclassified	6	–0.95	–1.12	–0.63
Unemployed	36	–0.74	–0.75	–0.35
Migration status of household head				
Indigenous	178	–0.88	–0.84	–0.34
Born in Accra—not indigenous	121	–0.75	–0.83	–0.44
Migrant	258	–0.91	–1.06	–0.63
Sex of head of household				
Male	362	–0.82	–0.91	–0.49
Female	195	–0.95	–0.99	–0.50

Source: Accra Study Team 1998.

fessions, business, or skilled labor have a higher nutritional status. Children in households with unemployed heads also appear to be somewhat better off, but the reason for this is not clear. Children from migrant families fare worse in terms of weight-for-age and weight-for-height measures than children from indigenous households or other households with heads born in Accra, but the association with height for age is not statistically significant. Gender of the head of the household is not associated with any of the nutritional status indicators.

Data from the Accra Urban Food and Nutrition study (AUFNS) survey (Accra Study Team 1998) were compared with data on the anthropometric status of Accra's children collected in a Demographic Health Survey (DHS) conducted in 1988 and another conducted by the government of Ghana in 1993 (GSS 1988 and 1993).[41]

[41] The study was designed so that the data collected would be comparable to the data from the DHSs of 1988 and 1993.

Table 38—Nutritional status data from AUFNS 1997 compared with 1988 and 1993 DHS data for children between 3 and 35 months

Measure	Source			Difference, 1988–93	Difference, 1993–97
	1988 DHS	1993 DHS	1998 AUFNS		
Z-score					
Mean anthropometric measurements					
Height-for-age (N = 151)					
Mean	–1.06	–0.64	–0.94	+.042	–0.30
[95% CI][a]	[–1.24– –0.88]	[–1.36– –1.04]	[–1.07– –0.81]	[0.15–0.70]	[–.054– –0.05]
Weight-for-age (N = 131)					
Mean	–1.20	–0.86	–1.05	+.034	–0.18
[95% CI][a]	[–1.36– –1.04]	[–1.05– –0.67]	[–1.17– –0.92]	[0.09–0.58]	[–0.41– +0.04]
Weight-for-height (N = 561)					
Mean	–0.64	–0.56	–0.57	+0.09	–0.01
[95% CI][a]	[–0.81– –0.48]	[–0.70– –0.41]	[–0.65–0.48]	[–0.13 +0.31]	[–0.18– +0.16]
Proportion					
Prevalence of malnutrition					
Stunted (height-for-age < –2) (N = 151)					
Percent	17.9	12.2	17.3	–36.0	+50.0
[95% CI][a]	[11.7–24.1]	[6.9–17.6]	[13.7–20.9]	[–67–+23]	[–14–+163]
Underweight (weight-for-age <–2)					
Percent	20.5	13.0	15.3	–42.0	+21.0
[95% CI][a]	[14.0–27.1]	[7.2–18.8]	[12.5–18.2]	[–70–+11]	[-31–+113]
Wasted (weight-for-height <–2)					
Percent	4.6	6.1	5.3	+34.0	–13.0
[95% CI][a]	[0.9–8.4]	[1.3–10.9]	[3.2–7.5]	[–59–+342]	[–66–+121]

Source: Accra Study Team 1998; GSS 1989;GSS 1994; GSS 1998.

Notes: AUFNS is the Accra Urban Food and Nutrition Survey; DHS is demographic and health survey. Intervals are corrected for design effects of sampling strategies. Enumeration areas in Accra were sampled first, then households within selected areas, leading to possible geographical homogeneity.

[a] CI = Confidence interval.

Nutritional data were available only for children age 3–36 months in the 1988 DHS survey and for children age 0–35 months in the 1993 survey. The comparison was therefore restricted to children age 3–35 months, a group for which all three surveys have comparable representative data.

Comparison of the mean anthropometrical indexes in the two surveys show that between 1988 and 1993 in Accra, mean height-for-age Z-scores in children age 3–35 months improved significantly (by 0.42 Z-scores) (Table 38). There was a parallel improvement in weight for age (one-third of a Z-score) but no evidence of a change in weight for height. Between 1993 and 1997, the earlier gains in height-for-age Z-scores were virtually reversed (a statistically significant drop of 0.3 Z-scores in average status). Changes in mean weight-for-age and weight-for-height Z-scores were not statistically significant over this period.

When data for the prevalence in malnutrition are compared, stunting (height for age less than –2 Z-scores) and underweight (weight for age less than –2 Z-scores) show the same pattern (Table 38). The prevalences decrease between 1988 and 1993, but these improvements are reversed (for stunting) or partially reversed (for underweight) between 1993 and 1997. However, none of the survey-to-survey changes in prevalence are statistically significant. The prevalence of wasting in Accra has been stable and low over the entire period (Figures 7 and 8).

Figure 7—Changes in anthropometry (mean Z-scores), 1988, 1993, and 1997 surveys

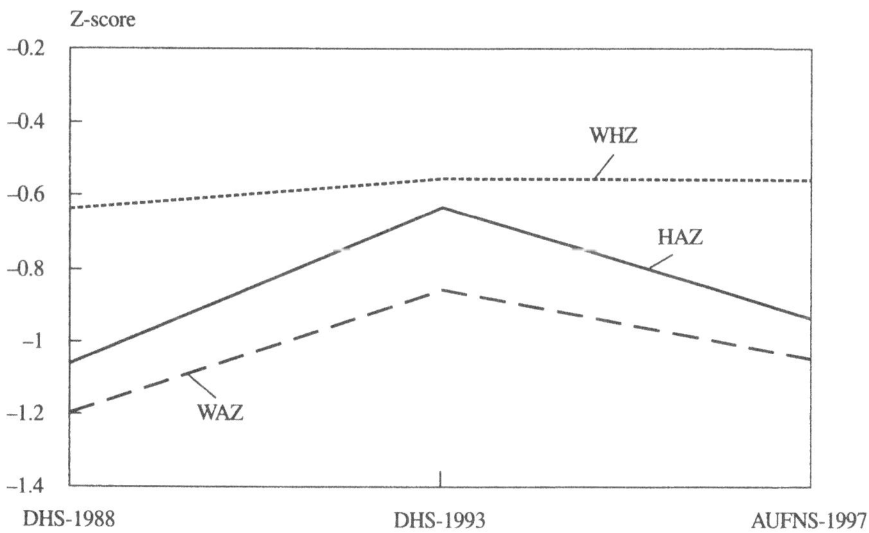

Sources: Accra Study Team 1998; GSS 1989; GSS 1994.
Notes: AUFNS is the Accra Urban Food and Nutrition Survey; DHS is demographic and health surveys.
HAZ is height-for-age Z-scores.
WAZ is weight-for-age Z-scores.
WHZ is weight-for-height Z-scores.

Figure 8—Changes in prevalence of malnutrition, 1988, 1993, and 1997 surveys

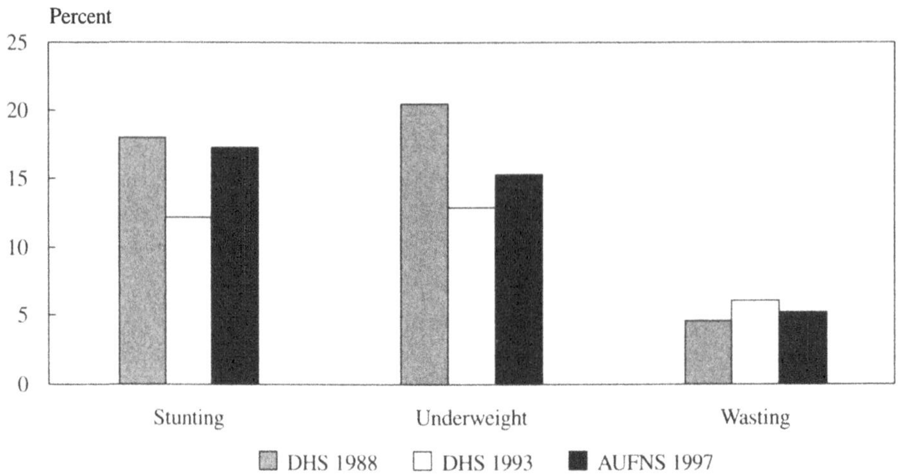

Sources: Accra Study Team 1998; GSS 1989; GSS 1994.

Notes: AUFNS is the Accra Urban Food and Nutrition Survey; DHS refers to demographic and health surveys conducted by the Government of Ghana in 1998 and 1993.

Stunting is below an anthropometric cut-off of –2 standard deviations below the median height-for-age Z-score. Underweight is below –2 standard deviations for weight-for-age Z-score. Wasting is below –2 standard deviations for weight-for-height Z-scores.

Health Status of Children

Visual Analog Scale

Researchers collected information on morbidity for the index child in each household, including the incidence of several common symptoms, and compiled a health visual analog score. The visual analog scale was used to collect information on mothers' perceptions of how their children's health compared with the health of other children the same age.[42] This measure is based on the assumption that mothers can accurately judge whether their children are generally sickly or healthy and is therefore somewhat subjective. The average health score was 71.30, with a standard deviation of 19.98. The distribution was skewed to the right, indicating that a larger proportion of mothers than would be expected in such a distribution considered their children healthier than other children of the same age. To correct for

[42] Visual analog scores for child and maternal health are based on the perception of primary caregivers. Caregivers were asked to compare their own and their children's health with that of their peers and their children's peers. Scores are based on a range of 0–100. Visual analog scales have been used for appetite ranking in Latin America and in developed countries (Stratton et al. 1998). For a complete description of the visual analog scale used in the present study, see Accra Study Team (1998).

Table 39—Index child morbidity

Characteristic	Frequency	Percent
Cough	267	47.8
Fever	205	36.7
Diarrhea	173	31.0
Difficult breathing	161	28.9
Vomiting	96	17.3
Rapid breathing	37	6.7

Source: Accra Study Team 1998.
Note: Symptoms are from the previous two weeks.

skewness, the scores were squared and divided by 100. This variable was used in all further analyses.

Short-Term Morbidity Symptoms

Mothers provided information on morbidity symptoms index children displayed in the two weeks before the survey (Table 39).[43] Approximately one-third of children had shown symptoms of diarrhea and 37 percent had developed fever. These prevalences are higher than those found for the greater Accra sample of the 1993 DHS, when both diarrhea and fever were approximately 16 percent.

These findings are not necessarily indicative of an increase in childhood morbidity between 1993 and 1997, because the differences could be largely the result of different sampling techniques or seasonal variations. Almost half the children in the sample were reported to have had a cough in the previous two weeks, and 29 percent had experienced "difficult breathing." The study considered difficult breathing a symptom of nasal congestion related to allergies, asthma, or mild upper respiratory infections. Rapid breathing was used as an indicator of severe lower respiratory infection and was prevalent among only 7 percent of the children. This prevalence is slightly lower than that reported in the 1993 DHS (9.7 percent), but the definition used in that survey included both coughing and rapid breathing.

Child Morbidity and Nutritional Status Indicators

The study found a lack of association between the health of children and their nutritional status (Table 40). Of all the morbidity symptoms studied, only fever in the previous two weeks was significantly associated with child nutritional status. The absence of strong associations reflects the fact that morbidity during the previous

[43] The information on morbidity was collected only on index children in the 0–36 month age group.

Table 40—Health and nutritional status of index child

	Number	Nutritional status (Z-scores)		
		Height-for-age	Weight-for-age	Weight-for-height
Illness during past two weeks				
Fever				
Yes	204	–1.01[a]	–1.06[a]	–0.55[a]
		(1.13)	(1.06)	(1.01)
No	352	–0.79	–0.87	–0.47
		(1.17)	(1.11)	(0.92)
Diarrhea				
Yes	172	–0.94[b]	–1.01[b]	–0.52[b]
		(1.13)	(1.02)	(0.92)
No	384	–0.83	–0.91	–0.49
		(1.17)	(1.12)	(0.97)
Cough				
Yes	265	–0.92[b]	–0.99[b]	–0.53[b]
		(1.12)	(1.13)	(0.93)
No	291	–0.82	–0.99	–0.46
		(1.14)	(1.05)	(0.97)
Vomiting				
Yes	95	–0.83[b]	–1.01[b]	–0.59[b]
		(1.08)	(0.96)	(0.84)
No	459	–0.80	–0.93	–0.48
		(1.18)	(1.12)	(0.97)
Difficult breathing				
Yes	161	–0.89[b]	–0.88[b]	–0.42[b]
		(1.22)	(1.16)	(0.92)
No	394	–0.86	–0.97	–0.53
		(1.14)	(1.06)	(0.96)
Rapid breathing				
Yes	36	–1.14[b]	–1.02[b]	–0.37[b]
		(1.06)	(1.22)	(1.11)
No	518	–0.85	–0.94	–0.50
		(1.17)	(1.08)	(0.94)
Index child's health analog				
<25th percentile		–1.32[a]	–0.74[a]	–1.17[a]
		(1.14)	(0.97)	(1.18)
25–50th percentile		–0.99	–0.56	–0.82
		(1.00)	(0.86)	(1.10)
50–75th percentile		–0.87	–0.43	–0.86
		(1.08)	(0.94)	(1.15)
75th percentile		–0.58	–0.23	–0.60
		(1.00)	(0.96)	(1.13)

Notes: Statistical significance of differences between groups was tested by t-test (two-group comparisons) and ANOVA (more than two groups comparison). Means are presented with standard deviations in parentheses.

[a] $p < 0.05$ (difference between groups considered statistically significant).

[b] $p \geq 0.05$ (difference between groups considered not statistically significant).

two weeks is not necessarily a good proxy for long-term morbidity. It is well recognized that long-term rather than short-term morbidity is likely to have a detectable negative impact on growth, particularly on stunting. Recent research has shown, for example, that every additional day of diarrhea increases the risk of subsequent mortality and poor weight gain (Morris et al. 1996). The health visual analog scale results in Table 40 do show a linear relationship with all three indicators of nutritional status, indicating that mothers' perception of their children's health is probably a more accurate proxy for long-term morbidity than symptoms experienced during the previous two weeks. Children rated by their mothers as having better-than-average health had significantly higher mean Z-scores for height for age, weight for age, and weight for height. The mean height-for-age score of children in the highest quartile of the health scale was 0.74 Z-scores greater than the mean score for children in the lowest quartile group.

Maternal Anthropometry and Health

Maternal average height, weight, and body mass index (BMI) were 160 centimeters, 63 kilograms, and 24 kilograms per meter squared (kg/m^2), respectively. Maternal stature was normally distributed, and only 3.2 percent of women were shorter than 149 centimeters—the cutoff that is often used to define obstetric risk (the likelihood of complications with childbirth). In general, short maternal stature is a much more severe problem in Asia and Latin America than in Africa (UN ACC/SCN 1992). The weight and BMI distributions were skewed to the right, indicating the presence of overweight and obese women among the sample. Some 36 percent of women had a BMI greater than or equal to 25, and 13 percent had a BMI greater than or equal to 30 kg/m^2. These results are not surprising, given that obesity has been described as an emerging problem among adults in many large urban areas in the developing world, including in Africa (Nago et al. 1996). At the other extreme, 10 percent of the women sampled had a BMI lower than 20, with 6 percent below 18.5 kg/m^2 (the cutoff points that are often used to define undernutrition in adults) (Gibson 1990). The DHS data from 1993 reported a similar prevalence of low BMIs (5.5 percent below 18.5 kg/m^2) among women from the Greater Accra region.

Health

A visual analog scale was also used with mothers, who were asked to evaluate their own health status and compare their health to that of other women their age. The average score was 71.56, with a standard deviation of 18.76. Like the distribution of the children's health scores, this one was skewed to the right. Mothers perceived themselves as generally healthy compared with other women the same age. The average age of mothers in the sample was 30 years old. As expected from this relatively young sample, the prevalence of reported chronic diseases was low: only 2 mothers reported having diabetes, 26 reported hypertension, 17 asthma, 18 heart illness, 17 anemia, and 6 arthritis.

Table 41—Prevalence of stunting in children with obese mothers (index children, 0–39 months old)

Maternal BMI	Number of mothers	Percent of mothers who are obese	Number of children stunted	Percent of children stunted
(kg/m^2)				
<20	86	15.7	15	17.4
20–24.9	262	47.8	41	15.6
25–26.9	62	11.3	9	14.5
≥27	138	25.2	20	14.5

Source: Accra Study Team 1998.
Note: BMI = body mass index. Obesity is BMI > 29 kg/m^2.

Overweight Mother/Stunted Child

During the qualitative community studies, researchers noted an apparently high prevalence of obese women and undernourished children in the same households, particularly in the indigenous neighborhoods of Accra (Ga Mashie Study Team 1996). In the perception of most respondents, this combination was the result of diet and livelihood activities (for the mothers) and poor childcare and inadequate food consumption (for the children). This phenomenon raises two important issues. The first involves its root cause. Do households allocate resources poorly and have poor caregiving practices, or is there an outright food security problem? The second point relates to the association between malnutrition in utero and during early childhood and the increased risk of chronic diseases during adult life (Barker 1994). Barker hypothesizes that a significant proportion of obese women living in poor urban areas of the developing world today were malnourished in utero and during early childhood. It is this group of women that may now be suffering some of the long-term negative consequences of early malnutrition (WHO 1997). This latter point could not be investigated in the present study because of a lack of information on the early childhood nutritional status of adult women in the sample.

In pursuing the first question, researchers compared the prevalence of children's stunting among four groups, using the mothers' BMIs (Gibson 1990). In the group of mothers with low BMIs (less than 20 kg/m^2), 17 percent of children were stunted, compared with approximately 14 percent in the group of mothers with BMIs greater than or equal to 27 kg/m^2 (Table 41). There were no differences in the prevalence of childhood stunting by maternal BMI, and the prevalence of stunting among underweight mothers was only slightly greater (the trend test was not statistically significant). These findings were confirmed using more extreme cutoff values (lower than 18.5 and higher than 30 kg/m^2).

These findings suggest that either maternal BMI is not a good proxy for household food availability in this population, or that food availability may not be the most important factor in the etiology of stunting in Accra. The next chapter will analyze the importance of other maternal and household factors.

CHAPTER 7

Caregiving Behaviors and Resources

Along with food security, the availability of health services, and a healthy environment, caregiving behaviors are one of the major determinants of good health and nutrition in young children. The analysis of care capacity at the household level takes into consideration a range of resources as well as the actual caregiving practices themselves. Care resources include human resources, as measured by maternal and household characteristics; economic resources available at the household level; and organization resources at both the household and the community level. Care behaviors are the actual practices that caregivers, households, and communities adopt to support the physical, mental, and social needs of the growing child and other household members. This chapter provides a descriptive analysis of *care resources,* particularly the characteristics of the principal caregiver (age, education, work status) and of the household (socioeconomic factors and the availability of services) that may affect the caregivers' ability to provide good care for the growing child. *Care behaviors* related specifically to child feeding, preventive health-seeking behavior, and hygiene are also reviewed. An analysis of the associations between these care resources and behavior is then presented, followed by an analysis of the associations between care behaviors and child nutritional status and morbidity outcomes.

Caregiving and Urbanization

The fact that this study took place in an urban setting deserves special mention, as the effects of urbanization may have serious consequences for care provision. Growing cities such as Accra are characterized by a deteriorating environment and physical infrastructure, a lack of basic services, an increased exposure to environmental contamination and rising poverty levels. Women, who are the primary care providers in most households, increasingly need to generate income. Nearly half of all females older than 10 years of age in this sample were engaged in income-generating activities in addition to their household responsibilities. Under such conditions, households can foster good health and nutrition in young children only if they can maximize the efficacy of use of their scarce resources.

Care Resources of Accra Households

Characteristics of Caregivers

In 96 percent of cases, the primary caregivers were the biological mothers of the index children. All but three of the caregivers who were not biological mothers were grandmothers. Data on care resources were collected on all primary caregivers, whether they were biological mothers or not, because personal and family characteristics influence all caring behaviors.

The majority of primary caregivers in the sample (63 percent) had some basic education. About 12 percent had no education at all, and 25 percent had a high school education or higher (Table 42). The predominant ethnic groups in the sample were the Ga and Adangbe, who are indigenous to the greater Accra region. About two-thirds of the primary caregivers were married and the only wife, while another 16 percent were single, either cohabiting or living alone. The majority of primary caregivers received some financial support from the father of their children.

The majority of primary caregivers were working, either full time (55 percent) or part time (9 percent). Of those working, 49 percent were selling in the markets or on the streets, 34 percent were working from home, and only 17 percent were either factory or office workers or shopkeepers. The large majority of primary caregivers took care of their children at all times (65 percent), and more than half looked after their child while working. The majority of primary caregivers worked in petty trading and street food vending, and many worked long hours (more than 8 hours per day). Some part of their activities took place at home, particularly in the most densely populated neighborhoods. At home, particularly in compound family houses, other people would be available to help with a kiosk or other small business and to look after the children, at least informally. On the streets or in the markets, this informal support would be less available. Only 35 percent of caregivers reported using some type of alternative childcare. Of those, the majority used a single person, 12 percent used more than one, and 28 percent used a crèche.

Household Care Resources

Other factors that may affect quality of caregiving—especially the caregivers' ability to maintain a hygienic environment—include the availability of water and sanitary facilities (see Chapter 3). The toilet facilities available to Accra's population are mainly public latrines (54 percent) and private improved pit latrines (20 percent). Only 10 percent of households had flush toilets at the time of the study, and 16 percent did not have or use any toilets at all (that is, they used empty lots and gutters). Sources of drinking water were mainly vendors or wells (54 percent). Only 38 percent of households had water in the compound of their homes, and just 7 percent had indoor piping. Waste disposal methods were mainly public dumping, dumping in gutters or empty lots, household's collection, and burying or burning on compounds of homes (Table 43).

Table 42—Characteristics of primary caregivers

Characteristic	Frequency	Percent
Education		
None	66	11.8
Some primary school	131	23.5
Some middle school or Islamic	98	17.6
Middle school graduate	122	21.9
Some secondary school	141	25.3
Migration status		
Indigenous	177	31.7
Not indigenous/born in Accra	152	27.2
Migrant	229	41.0
Ethnic origin		
Ga/Adangbe	203	36.4
Ashanti/Fanti/Akan	153	27.4
Ewe	132	23.7
Other	70	12.5
Marital status		
Single (cohabiting)	37	6.6
Single (not cohabiting)	51	9.1
Married (only wife)	373	66.8
Married (senior wife or other)	61	10.9
Separated, divorced, widowed	36	6.5
Receives financial support from children's father	434	77.8
Body Mass Index (kg/m^2)		
<20	86	15.7
20–24.9	261	47.7
25–26.9	62	11.3
≥27	138	25.2
Current employment		
Not working (not looking for work)	188	33.7
Working part time	53	9.5
Working full time	306	54.8
Unemployed (looking for work)	11	2.0
Place of employment		
Home	124	34.5
Markets/streets	175	48.7
Factory/office/shop	60	16.7
Usual hours worked per day		
Zero	150	28.6
0.5–3.5 hours	22	4.2
4–7.5 hours	146	27.9
≥8 hours	206	39.3
Alternate childcare		
Principal caregiver (cares for index child all the time)	361	65.3
Mother works and also looks after child	205	57.1
Childcare alternatives (N = 196):		
Single person	118	60.2
Multiple persons	23	11.7
Crèche	55	28.1
Age of alternate caretaker (N = 121)		
6–15 years old	15	12.4
16–49 years old	60	49.6
≥50 years old	46	38.0

Source: Accra Study Team 1998.
Note: N = 558.

Table 43—Water and sanitation facilities

Characteristics	Frequency	Percent
Toilet facilities		
None	91	16.3
Public latrine	299	53.6
Private improved pit latrine	113	20.3
Flush toilet	55	9.9
Source of drinking water		
Vendor/well	298	54.5
Piped outside	209	38.2
Piped inside	40	7.3
Waste disposal		
Gutter/empty lot/other	79	14.2
Bury/burn on compound	44	7.9
Public dumping bin	370	66.3
Household collection	65	11.6

Source: Accra Study Team 1998.
Notes: N = 558.

Care Behaviors of Primary Caregivers

The resources analyzed above are the factors that enable caregivers to provide care within the household. This section presents descriptive data on caring behaviors related to feeding, preventive health-seeking behaviors, and hygiene and describes the construction of two indexes, one for hygiene and another for care.

Breast-feeding and Complementary Feeding Practices

Breast-feeding is universal in most Ghanaian communities, both rural and urban. Rarely, however, do mothers follow current standard international recommendations to breast-feed infants exclusively for the first six months (Armar 1989; Ghana-MOH 1989; Armar-Klemesu 1998). In the sample, the moment when mothers initiated breast-feeding varied widely, ranging from 0 to 336 hours after birth, with a mean of 22 hours (Table 44). Only 19 percent of mothers initiated breast-feeding within the recommended hour of delivery, and up to 25 percent delayed breast-feeding for more than 24 hours after birth. Some 32 percent of mothers offered prelacteal feeds.

The median length of breast-feeding for mothers in the sample was 18.2 months. During the first four months, the majority of mothers gave their children a variety of complementary liquids and foods. The median age of inclusion of weaning foods in the children's diet was 5.2 months.[44] However, according to current recommendations

[44] These median ages were adjusted by survival analysis for truncated data—that is, cases where the practice had either not yet been started (such as the introduction of weaning food among young infants) or terminated (such as breast-feeding).

Table 44—Child feeding practices

Characteristics	Valid Number[a]	Frequency	Percent
Initiation of breast-feeding			
Mean number of hours after birth[b]	531	22.34 (38.08)	(Minimum 0, maximum 336)
Categories	531		
≤1 hour		100	18.8
2–5 hours		134	25.2
6–12 hours		94	17.7
13–24 hours		70	13.2
>24 hours		133	25.0
Prelacteal feeds			
Yes, given	530	180	32.4
Feeding 0–4 months	534		
Gave water		359	67.4
Gave sugared water		136	25.7
Gave infant formula		164	30.7
Gave milk		83	15.7
Gave solids/semisolids		217	40.6
Complementary feeding	557		
Gave special weaning food		478	85.8
Which special food?	475		
Koko		320	67.4
Cereal/infant formula		37	7.8
Weanimix/oats/custard		58	12.2
Mpotompoto/yam porridge		51	10.7
Soft *banku* stew		9	1.9
Who feeds the child?	557		
Primary caregiver		369	66.2
Other		40	7.2
No one		148	26.6
What is done when child refuses to eat?	552		
Use force		79	14.3
Coax/play with child		138	25.0
Change food		88	15.9
Leave child alone		112	20.3
Feel it's not a problem		135	24.5

Source: Accra Study Team 1998.

[a] Note that only biological mothers were asked questions related to the initiation of breast-feeding, use of prelacteal feeds, and child feeding practices between 0 and 4 months of age (N = 539). All other feeding practices were asked to the whole sample (N = 558), but sample sizes vary either because of truncated data (child not having reached the age yet) or true missing values.

[b] Standard deviation.

(WHO 1995; WHO 1998), complementary feeding should be introduced into children's diets starting around the age of 6 months. Special weaning foods are also recommended rather than the family diet. Young infants need soft foods and, more important they need foods that provide higher energy and nutrient density than most family diets provide. Even traditional weaning foods are often not ideal in terms of nutrient density (especially with regard to bioavailable vitamins and minerals). For this reason, many countries promote locally produced, cheap, and culturally acceptable fortified weaning mixtures.

In Ghana, *koko,* a thin, low-energy, low-nutrient porridge or gruel prepared from fermented maize dough, remains a popular traditional weaning food for infants. Consumption of *koko* was in fact implicated in the development of protein-energy malnutrition among Ghanaian children (Williams 1933). Efforts to encourage mothers to enrich the porridge by adding milk, fish powder, groundnut paste, or bean flour have been largely unsuccessful. To address this problem, since 1987 the Nutrition Division of Ghana's Ministry of Health, with support from UNICEF, has been promoting and encouraging the consumption of *weanimix,* a locally formulated cereal-legume mixture, as an alternative to *koko. Weanimix* has unfortunately not been widely accepted, and *koko* continues to be the preferred weaning food for the majority of Ghanaian infants (Armar-Klemesu 1996).

Some 86 percent of primary caregivers offered special weaning foods to the index child. *Koko* was the first food offered to the majority of children (67 percent), followed by *weanimix,* oats, or custard (12 percent), and by a porridge called *mpotompoto* (11 percent). The median age for the introduction of family food was 9.2 months. Primary caregivers fed children in 66 percent of cases, while 27 percent of children fed themselves and 7 percent were fed by an alternate caregiver. About 24 percent of mothers claimed that they had no problems feeding their children. But when children refused to eat, 14 percent of mothers reported trying to force them to eat, 25 percent tried coaxing or playing with the child, 16 percent tried another food, and 20 percent did nothing. Helping feed and stimulate children during meals is recognized as an important component of psychosocial care, especially for children with poor appetites (Bentley, Black, and Hurtado 1995).

Preventive Health-Seeking Behaviors

Health-seeking behaviors include both the management of illness at home—prevention, diagnosis, and treatment—and the utilization of health services. Only the preventive use of health services for mothers and index children were addressed in this study, however.

Almost all mothers (97 percent) had attended prenatal care at some point during their pregnancies—the same results found for urban mothers in the 1993 DHS (the figure was 84 percent in rural areas). But about half of the women in this survey sought prenatal care only during their second trimester, and a small proportion waited until the third trimester or just before birth (Table 45). Mothers reported that

Table 45—Health-seeking behaviors

Characteristics	Frequency	Percent
Mother attended prenatal care[a]	518	97.2
When was the first time?		
First trimester	232	44.5
Second trimester	262	50.3
Third trimester	21	4.0
Just before birth	6	1.2
Mother took the following in the last month:		
Antimalarial prophylaxis	124	22.2
Deworming medication	38	6.8
Vitamin supplements	116	20.8
Iron supplements	111	19.9
Mother gave the child the following in the last month:		
Antimalarial prophylaxis	291	52.2
Deworming medication	105	18.8
Vitamin supplements	223	40.0
Mother took the child for		
Growth monitoring	357	64.0
DPT immunization (n = 513)[b]	463	90.3
Measles immunization (n = 392)[b]	338	86.2

Source: Accra Study Team 1998.
Note: N = 558.
[a] This question was asked only of biological mothers (N = 553)
[b] For diphtheria, pertussis, and tetanus (DPT) immunization, the sample includes only children older than 3 months, and for measles, the sample includes children older than 9 months (ages at which these two immunizations are expected to be completed).

both they and their children used antimalarial drugs, deworming medication, and vitamin and mineral supplements. But qualitative research showed that these medications and supplements were used for curative rather than preventive purposes.

During the month preceding the survey, 64 percent of children had been taken for growth monitoring, and most had been immunized for diphtheria, pertussis, and tetanus (DPT) and measles. Urban areas typically have much higher rates of immunization coverage than rural areas (Ruel et al. 1998). Attendance at growth monitoring was higher among smaller infants (less than 9 months old), suggesting that attendance was probably motivated by the immunization schedule.

Hygiene Behaviors

Hygiene practices directly affect the cleanliness of the environment and the number of infectious agents children ingest, either through contaminated food or water or by placing contaminated objects in their mouths. Researchers measured hygiene behaviors using a spot-check method. Fieldworkers were trained to observe and grade a list of 11 hygiene-related aspects of each caregiver and index

Table 46—Frequency of good hygiene behaviors

Observation	Households with good hygiene		Number of missing/not observed
	(number)	(percent)	
Primary caregiver clean[a]	388	70.2	6
Index child clean[a]	389	71.0	11
Diaper clean[a]	383	70.5	16
Compound swept	273	50.0	13
No poultry feces[a]	369	69.9	31
No stagnant water[a]	487	89.4	14
No garbage in compound	340	74.4	102
No unwashed utensils	293	70.8	145
Drinking water covered	105	68.6	406
House swept	226	79.0	273
No human feces	522	97.8	25

Source: Accra Study Team 1998.
Note: Based on observations made during a hygiene spot check.
[a] Indicates variables used in the hygiene index.

child as well as their house and compound (Table 46). This method is generally used in cross-sectional surveys that do not allow researchers to carry out day-long observations in the homes. The elements of the spot check are proxies for good or bad behaviors—for instance, whether the compound was swept or the mother's hands were clean. Field workers did not have to observe the behaviors themselves—that is, they did not have to see the mother sweeping the compound or washing her hands frequently.[45]

Creating the Hygiene and Care Indexes

The Hygiene Index. This index was constructed using the hygiene variables that had fewer than 100 missing or unobserved data and for which the data showed sufficient variability (the first six variables in Table 46).[46] Each positive behavior (for example, compound swept) received a value of 1, and each negative behavior (for example, compound not swept) was assigned a value of 0. The variables were the cleanliness of the primary caregiver, index child, and index child's diaper; whether the compound was swept; and the absence of poultry feces and stagnant water in

[45] Training and standardizing fieldworkers well is key to the success of this methodology. The observations are generally subjective, and fieldworkers have to agree on what constitutes "clean" and "dirty," what is swept and what is not, and how many flies are "a lot of flies." Researchers paid careful attention to these issues.

[46] One variable was found to have too little variability to be included in the index—"presence of human feces in the compound," which was 0 in 98 percent of the sample.

[47] Due to missing values in a number of variables used to create the index, the sample size for this index was 512.

the compound.[47] The index was the sum of the six variables, and scores ranged from 0 to 6.

Based on the frequency distribution of the index, three categories of hygiene practices were created:

1. Bad—those with scores of 0–3 (30.3 percent);
2. Average—those with scores of 4–5 (39.5); and
3. Good—those with the maximum score (6) (30.3).

The Care Index. No single indicator can capture the complex patterns of behavior that constitute good child care. Researchers therefore created a care index to reflect the combination of factors measured in this study, using data on child feeding practices and the use of preventive health care services (Table 47).[48] The general principle was to allocate a score of –1 for a practice believed to be harmful, 0 for a practice believed to be beneficial, and +1 for a particularly beneficial practice. Practices were considered beneficial or harmful based on current child feeding recommendations (WHO 1995; WHO 1998) and on available scientific evidence about the benefits or risks of these practices.

The index was made age specific so that both the variables and scoring system could vary by age as appropriate. Scores for the different practices were then added up to create the index for each age group. The maximum possible score for each group was +2, and the minimum was –11. The mean and standard deviations were –2.49 and 1.91, respectively. Terciles were created to form three categories of overall caring practices—poor, average, and good.

Associations Between Care Resources and Care Practices

According to the conceptual model (Figure 2), care resources have a direct effect on caring behaviors, which in turn are important determinants of children's nutritional and health status. This section uses bivariate analysis to examine how care resources are related to care practices in the sample.

Of all the factors studied at either level (individual primary caretaker or household), only the formal education of the primary caregiver is associated positively with both the care and hygiene indexes (Table 48). Household expenditure levels are not associated with the care index in these bivariate analyses, but they are positively associated with good hygiene. Maternal working status, number of hours worked, and use of alternate childcare are not significantly related to either index. The association found between place of work and the hygiene score probably reflects differences in socioeconomic status between primary caregivers who work in

[48] The index was created only for children 4 months or older, because only two variables (the first two in Table 47) were available to construct the index for infants below this age. This adjustment brought the sample size to 512 children. Owing to missing values in some of the variables included in the index, the final sample size was 475 children.

Table 47—Practices and scoring system used, by age group, to create the care index (for children 4–36 months old)

Care practice	Scores allocated to different practices, by age group (months)		
	4–8.9	9–17.9	≥18
Scores for breast-feeding and feeding practices			
Prelacteal feeds used	Yes:–1 No: 0	Yes:–1 No: 0	Yes:–1 No: 0
Still breast-feeding	No =–1 Yes = 1	No = 0 Yes = 1	
Gave water to child 0–4 months old	Yes:–1 No: 0	Yes:–1 No: 0	Yes:–1 No: 0
Gave sugar-based liquids to child 0–4 months old	Yes:–1 No: 0	Yes:–1 No: 0	Yes:–1 No: 0
Gave infant formula to child 0–4 months old	Yes:–1 No: 0	Yes:–1 No: 0	Yes:–1 No: 0
Gave cow's milk to child 0–4 months old	Yes:–1 No: 0	Yes:–1 No: 0	Yes:–1 No: 0
Gave solid foods to child 0–4 months old	Yes:–1 No: 0	Yes:–1 No: 0	Yes:–1 No: 0
First food offered to child			
Unfortified cereals (*koko*)	0	0	0
Fortified cereals	+1	+1	+1
No special weaning foods	–1	–1	–1
Does anyone help the child eat?		No: –1 Yes: 0	No: –1 Yes: 0
What does caregiver do when child refuses to eat?			
Nothing (child left alone)	–1	–1	–1
Other (coax, play with, force, change food, not a problem)	0	0	0
Preventive health care services used			
Growth monitoring (past month)	No: –1 Yes: 0	No: –1 Yes: 0	No: –1 Yes: 0
DPT immunization (>3 months)	No: –1 Yes: 0	...	...
Measles immunization (>9 months)	...	No: –1 Yes: 0	No: –1 Yes: 0

Source: Accra Study Team 1998.
Note: DPT = diphtheria, pertussis, and tetanus.

the markets and streets and those who work in shops, factories, and offices. No association was found between the age, nutritional, or health status of the primary caregiver and care or hygiene practices scores. Although these findings are tentative because they do not control for any potential confounding factors, they tend to confirm the overwhelming importance of maternal schooling for all aspects of childcare.

Table 48—Association between care resources and care practices

Care resource	Care index (n = 475) Number	Care index (n = 475) Mean score	Care index (n = 475) Standard deviation	Hygiene index (n = 512) Number	Hygiene index (n = 512) Percent with 0–3 good practices	Hygiene index (n = 512) Percent with 6 good practices
Characteristics of primary caregiver						
Education						
None	53	–3.00*	(1.71)	63	44.4*	28.6
Primary to middle school	297	–2.56	(1.88)	322	32.0	24.8
Some secondary school	125	–2.08	(1.98)	127	18.9	44.9
Employment status						
Does not work (not seeking work)	143	–2.17	(1.88)	176	25.6	36.4
Works part time	48	–2.50	(1.81)	52	26.9	36.5
Works full time	274	–2.63	(1.90)	275	33.5	25.1
Looking for work	10	–3.10	(2.56)	9	44.4	33.3
Workplace						
Home	109	–2.60	(1.75)	117	32.5*	24.8
Markets/streets	159	–2.65	(1.90)	158	40.5	21.5
Shop/factory/office	54	–2.50	(2.11)	52	7.7	48.1
Cares for child all the time						
Yes	294	–2.43	(1.88)	339	28.9	30.4
No	176	–2.64	(1.93)	169	32.5	30.2
Takes child to work						
Yes	179	–2.65	(1.86)	193	31.1	24.9
No	143	–2.56	(1.91)	134	34.3	29.9
Type of childcare alternative						
Single caregiver	110	–2.50	(1.83)	108	35.2	27.8
Multiple caregiver	20	–2.20	(2.09)	18	55.6	16.7
Crèche	50	–2.92	(2.16)	46	19.6	41.3
Number of hours usually worked						
0	117	–2.37	(1.88)	278	28.1	34.2
½–3½ hours	120	–2.48	(1.98)	25	44.0	20.0
4–7½ hours	131	–2.66	(1.86)	86	31.4	24.4
≥8 hours	179	–2.61	(1.99)	123	31.7	27.6
Household characteristics						
Expenditure quintile						
1	95	–2.62	(1.85)	104	46.2*	18.3
2	93	–2.53	(1.93)	103	36.9	31.1
3	94	–2.68	(1.80)	100	27.0	26.0
4	99	–2.35	(1.91)	101	27.7	30.7
5	93	–2.27	(2.05)	102	13.7	46.1

Source: Accra Study Team 1998.

* $p < 0.05$ (results of ANOVA for care index, and of chi^2 test for hygiene index).

Table 49—Care index and nutritional status: Health outcomes for children 4–36 months old

Care index (tercile)	Number	Height for age	Weight for age	Weight for height	Health score[a]
1	145	–1.18*	–1.29*	–0.71	48.22*
		(1.27)	(1.08)	(0.91)	(26.00)
2	180	–0.89	–0.99	–0.51	55.84
		(1.11)	(1.06)	(0.92)	(24.43)
3	150	–0.66	–0.85	–0.52	58.90
		(1.03)	(0.97)	(0.99)	(23.16)

Source: Accra Study Team 1998.
Note: N = 475.
[a] Results of visual analog scale, squared.
* $p < 0.05$ (results of ANOVA test).

Association between Care Practices and Child Nutrition and Health Outcomes

Better caregiving practices were associated with a better nutritional status, as reflected by higher mean height-for-age and weight-for-age Z-scores and a lower prevalence of stunted and underweight children (Table 49 and Figure 9). The magnitude of the difference in Z-scores for children whose primary caretaker scored in

Figure 9—The association between maternal care practices (terciles) and malnutrition prevalence

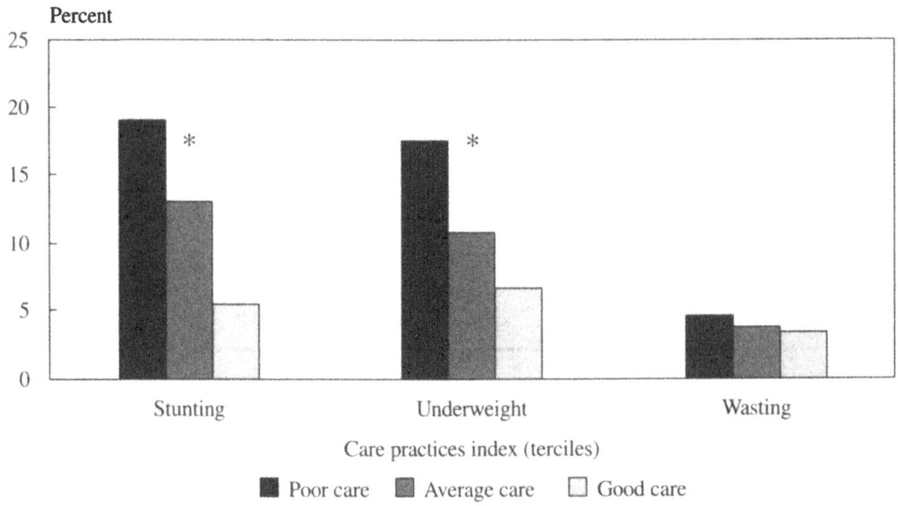

Source: Accra Study Team 1998.
* Statistically significant difference ($p < 0.05$).

Table 50—Hygiene index by child anthropometry and health score (visual analog scale)

Value	N[a]	Height-for-age Z-score[b]	Weight-for-age Z-score	Weight-for-height Z-score	Health score[c]
0–3 good practices	155	–1.07*	–1.11*	–0.57	51.34*
		(1.08)	(1.04)	(0.93)	(26.63)
4 or 5 good practices	200	–0.81	–0.85	–0.42	52.45
		(1.27)	(1.16)	(0.96)	(25.25)
6 good practices	155	–0.68	–0.85	–0.51	61.19
		(1.01)	(1.00)	(0.91)	(22.01)

[a] N = 512. Two values were missing in anthropometry, reducing the sample size to 510.
[b] Means and standard deviations are presented (in parenthesis).
[c] Results of visual analog scale, squared.
*$p < 0.05$ (results of ANOVA test).

the worst care tercile (1) and those for children whose primary caretaker scored in the best (3) is around 0.5 Z-scores for both height for age and weight for age. Better care practices were associated with dramatically lower levels of stunting (24.1 percent versus 7.3 percent) and underweight (22.1 percent versus 8.7 percent). There was no association with wasting or with mean weight-for-height Z-scores. However, this fact is not surprising, considering that wasting is not a major nutritional problem in this population (it has an overall prevalence of 5.3 percent).

The reported prevalence of diarrhea in the previous two weeks was not significantly associated with the care index, but fever was. Children whose primary caregiver scored in the lowest care tercile had a reported prevalence of fever of 46 percent, compared with 38 percent among children of caregivers in the highest care tercile (these results are not shown). As expected, good hygiene practices were significantly associated with a lower prevalence of diarrhea in the previous two weeks and with higher mean height-for-age and weight-for-age Z-scores, but there was no association with weight-for-height scores or with wasting (Tables 50 and 51).

Table 51—Hygiene index by whether child had diarrhea or fever in past two weeks

Hygiene index tercile	Had diarrhea		Had fever	
	Number[a]	Percent	Number[a]	Percent
0–3 good practices	61	39.4*	60	38.7
4 or 5 good practices	60	29.7	75	37.1
6 good practices	36	23.2	50	32.3

[a] N = 512. Two values were missing in anthropometry, reducing the sample size to 510.
*$p < 0.05$ (results of chi^2 test).

These findings confirm that care practices related to child feeding, use of preventive health care, and hygiene are important to children's nutritional status and health. Hygiene appears to have a more direct effect on infectious diseases and thus indirectly affects growth, especially in the long term. Feeding practices (at least the practices studied) may have a more direct effect on nutritional status and growth, but they may also have an effect on infectious diseases through appetite and immunity. Hygiene is strongly associated with the prevalence of diarrhea, but care is not. Hygiene and care are associated with mean height-for-age and weight-for-age Z-scores.

Other Factors Affecting Care

Life in urban areas is thought to present special challenges for the provision of adequate care, as noted earlier. The trade-offs women face between their productive and reproductive roles are likely to be more acute in urban than rural areas. Women in urban areas are often thought to be more likely than women in rural areas to work outside the home, for instance. According to the 1993 DHS data, however, this notion does not hold true in Ghana, where 50.7 percent of women in rural areas and 43.4 percent in urban areas work outside the home. But in this sample from Accra, about two-thirds of all primary caregivers of young children engaged in some kind of income-generating activity. The majority of them worked at a location away from their homes, and a large plurality of them worked very long hours. In spite of their apparently heavy workloads, up to two-thirds of primary caregivers cared for their children at all times. Among those who worked, more than half still looked after their child on a full-time basis. Only 35 percent of households reported using some type of alternative childcare.

Bivariate analysis does not show any association between maternal work patterns and childcare practices. This finding may be due to the fact that mothers do continue to take care of their child while they work and thus are able to breast-feed and take care of infants' special needs. Qualitative results, which Chapter 10 explores in greater detail, reveal that mothers of young children perceive that work can limit their ability to provide adequate childcare. At the same time, these women know that they must earn an income in order to provide food and other necessities for their children. Results here suggest that many working women are able to cope with this dilemma (see Chapter 9).

The next chapter examines the possible links between health and nutrition and the communities where people live, as well as the implications for targeting programs if neighborhoods are found to be mixed rather than homogeneous (Morris et al. 1999).

CHAPTER 8

Spatial Clustering of Outcomes

Earlier studies of Accra have characterized entire neighborhoods homogeneously in terms of ethnicity, density, centrality, and income and have relied on these characterizations for policy recommendations (Housing and Urban Development Associates 1990; Ghana—MLG 1992; Benneh et al. 1993; Songsore and McGranahan 1993).[49] Certainly, there are valid reasons for presuming some degree of spatial homogeneity in terms of income and therefore in measures of human welfare in Accra. Findings from this study, however, suggest that neighborhoods in Accra are more mixed than was previously assumed. This finding has important implications for future studies and interventions in the city.

Accra's neighborhoods have generally been perceived as homogeneous for several reasons. First, the underlying process of urbanization in Accra has resulted in sharp contrasts between indigenous and migrant neighborhoods. These differences give rise to cultural singularities in household composition and structure, as well as in child-raising practices. In indigenous neighborhoods in particular, many people live in family-compound houses and do not pay rent, as noted in Chapter 5—a factor that tends to limit their ability to change residences.

Second, other patterns of residence tend to promote less mobility within the city. The cost of rent and the tendency of landlords to demand several years' rent in advance promote greater income differentiation at the neighborhood level and reduce short-term mobility (in place of residence, at least). Third, there are major differences in human capital and housing quality (including housing density)—factors known to affect health and nutrition outcomes—in the city's neighborhoods. And finally, neighborhood infrastructure, including services, programs, and community development projects, may directly affect health and nutrition outcomes in certain areas of the city.

The presence or absence of significant spatial homogeneity in outcomes related to poverty and poor health and nutrition is an important factor in planning poverty alleviation programs or infrastructure projects. Beneficiaries must have a high

---

[49] While the size of these neighborhoods varies considerably, on average they are 7–8 times larger than the enumeration areas delineated by the GSS that were used for this survey.

Table 52—Welfare measures, by enumeration area

Enumeration area	Housing asset environment index[a]	Total per capita household expenditure[a]	Proportion of expenditure spent on food	Proportion of live-born children died
		(1,000 cedis)	(percent)	(percent)
Pokoase	–0.39	664	58.0	11.9
Dansoman	1.75	1,757	39.0	1.6
Korle Gonno	0.19	767	57.1	9.4
Lartebiokorshie	0.34	1,043	47.0	7.5
Odorkor	0.13	819	52.2	7.7
Bubiashie	0.43	1,002	51.3	8.7
Jamestown	–0.20	779	55.1	9.6
Osu	0.11	841	59.4	6.6
Adabraka	0.38	989	56.3	6.3
Teshie	–0.30	735	60.0	11.6
Labadi	0.04	760	53.2	5.1
Nima	–0.46	699	56.8	16.3
Accra New Town	–0.16	740	53.2	7.1
Maamobi	–0.21	792	55.3	7.5
Tema New Town	–1.42	547	61.9	13.0
Ashaiman	–0.09	698	54.9	5.9
P-value	<0.001	<0.001	<0.001	0.113

[a] An index of quality of housing, assets, and environmental quality was created based on four assets: refrigerator, electric stove, tape deck, and television set. Factor analysis was then used to derive one factor that would summarize variables related to the quality of housing (construction material for roof, walls, and floor), the "possession" index, the source of drinking water, and the availability of sanitary facilities and garbage disposal. The principal components factor extraction method was used. Loadings smaller than 0.5 were excluded from the initial model. The final model had five variables (floor, walls, water source, possession index, and sanitary facilities), all with factor loadings greater than 0.53, and explained 46 percent of the variance.

[b] Geometric mean.

probability of being truly needy (that is, the screening mechanism must demonstrate a high *positive predictive value*) and nonbeneficiaries a correspondingly low probability of being truly needy (the screening mechanism must show a high *negative predictive value*). Interventions using neighborhood targeting that is reasonably efficient in locating the truly needy could be much less expensive than interventions targeting households or individuals.

The data presented in Table 52 tests whether such geographic targeting is feasible in Accra. In particular, the distributions of the following measures are examined for evidence of homogeneity in the survey's 16 enumeration areas:

- An index of housing assets and environment (see notes to Table 52);
- Total per capita household expenditure and the proportion of the household budget allocated to food (Chapter 5);
- The proportion of children of the index child's principal caregiver that were born alive but have subsequently died;

Table 53—Nutrition and health measures, by enumeration area

	Internally standardized Z-scores			Health visual analog scores	
Enumeration area	Height for age	Weight for age	Weight for height	Caregiver	Index child
Pokoase	0.13	0.09	0.04	47.7	37.8
Dansoman	0.68	0.60	0.29	60.5	68.4
Korle Gonno	–0.12	–0.10	0.04	49.9	50.9
Lartebiokorshie	0.27	0.29	0.16	59.7	61.3
Odorkor	–0.20	–0.22	–0.11	53.4	55.8
Bubiashie	–0.19	–0.05	0.15	54.7	56.6
Jamestown	–0.16	–0.08	0.02	50.9	62.3
Osu	–0.11	–0.11	–0.03	56.7	59.7
Adabraka	0.29	0.25	0.08	55.0	49.8
Teshie	–0.26	–0.22	–0.01	52.0	48.3
Labadi	0.19	0.25	0.21	55.9	59.7
Nima	–0.04	–0.05	–0.05	55.1	52.6
Accra New Town	–0.10	–0.49	–0.52	65.8	58.1
Maamobi	–0.04	–0.05	0.00	53.0	58.2
Tema New Town	0.06	0.20	0.23	56.1	54.1
Ashaiman	0.00	–0.19	–0.27	49.6	43.6
P-values	0.026	0.008	0.153	0.243	<0.001

Source: Accra Study Team 1998.

- The anthropometric status of children under five years—height for age, weight for age, and weight for height (Chapter 6); and
- The perceived morbidity of the index child and the caregiver (the visual analog scores described in Chapter 6).

The housing index, expenditures, and food budget share all differed significantly across the 16 clusters (P = <0.001) (Table 52).[50] The proportion of children born alive that had died before the time of the survey did not differ significantly across clusters.

Table 53 shows the anthropometric status of children under five years (internally standardized Z-scores[51]) and the perceived health status of index children and their principal caregivers.[52] Height-for-age and weight-for-age Z-scores both differed significantly across clusters, but weight for height did not. Similarly, the perceived morbidity of the index child differed significantly across clusters, but the perceived morbidity of the caregiver did not. Table 54 shows, for the same nine measures of

[50] The expenditure variable was log-transformed prior to analysis to reduce the asymmetry in its distribution.

[51] Internally standardized Z-scores are used in this analysis, since those factors that affect the anthropometric status of *all* children in the sample, including defects of the WHO/NCHS growth standard, are not relevant to issues of intraurban differentials.

[52] The visual analog scores for the morbidity of both child and caregiver were squared and divided by 100 prior to analysis to reduce the asymmetry in their distributions.

Table 54—Variability between and within clusters

Item	Estimated between-E.A. Standard Deviation	Estimated within-E.A. Standard Deviation	Estimated within-E.A. correlation
Housing assets and environment index	0.60	0.80	0.38*
Log total per capita household expenditure	0.23	0.58	0.14*
Proportion of total household expenditure spent on food	4.63	15.42	0.09*
Internally standardized height-for-age Z-score	0.19	1.04	0.03*
Internally standardized weight-for-age Z-score	0.20	1.06	0.04*
Internally standardized weight-for-height Z-score	0.10	1.01	0.01
Perceived morbidity of index child's principal caregiver[a]	1.89	23.94	0.01
Perceived morbidity of index child	6.14	24.09	0.06*
Proportion of live-born children that have died	...	...	0.02

Note: E.A. = enumeration area.
[a] The original Visual Analog Scale measures were approximately normalized by squaring and dividing by 100.
* Significantly different from zero at the 5 percent level.

welfare described above, the estimated standard deviations within and among clusters and the estimated correlation coefficients within clusters.[53]

The findings presented in Table 54 show that for all nine variables examined, variability was considerably higher within clusters than across them. This effect was especially marked for the nutrition and health indicators. As a result, within-cluster correlations tend to be small and in some cases not significantly different from zero. These cases include weight for height, morbidity of the index child's principal caretaker, and mortality of previously living children. Only the housing asset and environment index showed evidence of nonnegligible within-cluster correlation (ρ = 0.38). For per capita expenditures, the within-cluster correlation fell from 0.14 to just below 0.10 when the 11 households with annual per capita expenditures greater than ₡4 million were excluded from the analysis.

Implications of the Findings

These results indicate a remarkable level of mixing within the enumeration areas sampled in the survey. Although the quality of the housing showed a certain degree

[53] For all variables except child mortality, estimates are by random-effects analysis of variance (see note to Table 52), based on the assumption that the actual children in the sample are intended merely to represent all possible living children in the cluster. For child mortality, which is not a continuous variable but rather a proportion estimated at the household level, the analysis of the variance cannot be used without violating the model's assumptions. The within-cluster correlation was therefore estimated using the semi-parametric Generalized Estimating Equation approach (Liang and Zeger 1986).

of uniformity at the cluster level, the families living in these houses had very different income levels and health outcomes. For example, all 16 enumeration areas included at least one household in the highest income quintile, while 14 had at least one household in the lowest quintile. The levels of homogeneity within clusters are comparable to those found in previous studies of rural areas, at least for mortality and general morbidity (Bennett et al. 1991). Deaton (1997) reports that rural areas of developing countries frequently show correlations for consumption in the range of 0.3–0.4.

Higher within-cluster correlations of welfare measures were expected in this representative sample of Accra because of the visible differences in low-income indigenous, low-income migrant, and modern middle-class neighborhoods. The relatively small number of clusters sampled may have resulted in a low (but consistent and unbiased) estimate of the true variances among clusters and thus also the correlation coefficients within clusters. However, this underestimation would have to be very substantial to reverse the conclusion that cluster-level effects are much less significant than individual- and household-level effects for health and nutrition outcomes in Accra.

This finding suggests that virtually all of the variation in income in Accra, as well as health and nutrition outcomes, is explained by factors that vary at the household and individual levels and not by community-level effects. Therefore, analysis and intervention must focus primarily on households and individuals, although possible interactions between variables at these levels and community-level variables must also be evaluated. The mixed nature of Accra's neighborhoods also has major implications for targeting strategies. Large-scale programs aiming to reach the greatest number of people in need while excluding the better-off cannot do so by operating in a few select neighborhoods. Rather, targeting strategies must be developed that reach the poor or vulnerable wherever they may reside. The Appendix describes some of the alternative targeting indicators that grew out of this study.

CHAPTER 9

Multivariate Determinants of Food Security, Health, Care, and Nutritional Status

The previous chapters have used a variety of qualitative and quantitative methods to determine the main constraints to achieving good child nutrition in Accra. This chapter complements those analyses with a multivariate regression investigation of the determinants of child nutritional status.

As in previous chapters, the conceptual framework presented in Chapter 1 (Figure 2) guides the multivariate analysis by identifying the multiple and complex pathways through which various factors affect nutritional status. Income follows one such pathway: high income provides household food security and high calorie intake, leading to good nutrition. Numerous studies have explored the link between income and nutritional status (Sahn 1994; see Strauss and Thomas 1995 for a review of these).[54] Income opens also a second important pathway, improving nutrition by raising the demand for nonfood inputs (goods and services) to health. Maternal education follows a similar pathway, increasing women's caregiving resources and improving childcare practices. Few studies have looked at care practices as an input into nutritional status, however (Haddad et al. 1996; Kumar, Naved, and Bhattarai 1997; Ruel et al. 1998). This investigation is unusual in that it does incorporate care practices into an otherwise standard regression approach.

The analysis uses regression techniques to identify the key constraints to good child nutrition in Accra, building on the bivariate analysis of previous chapters. The underlying model described in this section examines the pathways suggested by the conceptual model to explore the factors associated with good nutritional outcomes. The inputs of primary interest are household food availability, care, and health. Since

[54] Alderman and Garcia (1993) and Strauss and Thomas (1995) review the debate on the responsiveness of calorie intake to changes in income. Many studies also use measures of illness, including the incidence of diarrhea or the number of days ill, as a predictor of nutritional status (Alderman 1990; Cebu Study Team 1992). See Haddad et al. (1996) for a review of other studies.

each of these is also determined by a number of factors, each will be analyzed individually and in relation to nutritional status.

The Basic Model for the Empirical Approach

The theoretical model underpinning the econometric approach is the standard unitary household model. The data may reject this model because of the diversity of household types found during the qualitative analysis. However, it was difficult to identify a particular nonunitary or collective model that would be appropriate for all households. Thus the model controls for the possibility of heterogeneity in intrahousehold allocation rules by using ethnicity and headship variables.

The model for nutritional status is derived from the household production models. The household maximizes the joint utility function, which comprises the health and nutrition of each household member, goods purchased and produced at home, and leisure (Behrman and Deolalikar 1988; Strauss and Thomas 1995). Since the focus is on the index child's nutritional status, the utility function is expressed as

$$U = U(H_i, C_i, L_i),$$

where

H_i is the nutritional status of the index child i (measured by the standardized anthropometric measurement of height for age),

C_i is the consumption of goods, and

L_i is leisure.

H_i is an outcome of the height production function,

$$H_i = f(X_i, X_h, X_d, X_c, \mu),$$

where

X_i is a set of exogenous child-specific characteristics,

X_h is a set of exogenous household-specific characteristics,

X_d is a vector of endogenous household-specific inputs,

X_c is a set of exogenous community-specific variables, and

μ represents unobserved heterogeneity.

The input vector X_d represents outcomes of livelihood security that are inputs into nutritional status. A number of inputs were identified from the conceptual framework presented in Chapter 1 (Figure 2). Data limitations prevent the exploration of all of these, so that the focus is on the three most important factors influencing nutritional status: food, care, and health. Each input demand function can be represented as follows:

$$X_d = g(Y, Z, \mu),$$

where Y is a vector of exogenous household characteristics, and Z is a vector of endogenous variables.

Econometric Specification and Issues

The focus on household food availability, care, and child health as proximate determinants of child nutrition status poses problems for the regression analysis. These inputs into nutritional status are also outcomes of a variety of factors, one of which is income. An ordinary least squares (OLS) estimation of a regression with nutrition as an outcome and these three proximate variables as determinants could be biased for two reasons. First, there may be unobserved variables that are relegated to the error term but are correlated with the variables included on the right side. Second, explanatory variables may exist that are endogenous to or codetermined with the outcome variable and hence are correlated with the error term.

The typical approach to dealing with the first problem is a fixed-effects estimation at the community, household, or individual level. Since the data are cross-sectional, only community fixed effects can be used. The second approach to addressing these problems is to use instrumental variables (IV). The credibility of the IV approach rests on the ability to find variables that are correlated with the suspected endogenous explanatory variables but that do not affect the outcome variable (other than through the explanatory variable being instrumented). This approach requires finding a variable that can affect household food consumption but not malnutrition. The task is difficult and challenging, especially when there are three explanatory variables to instrument. Few other researchers have faced this challenge (Haddad et al. 1996).

The multivariate analysis estimates a system of four equations explaining

1. household calorie availability,
2. health of the index child,
3. care behaviors and practices used by the primary caregiver of the index child, and
4. standardized height for age of the index child.

These equations are estimated using IV, employing the appropriate tests to determine the credibility of the approach. In general, OLS estimates will be inconsistent in the presence of an endogenous variable on the right side. IV estimates are consistent but less efficient. However, they can be biased if the selected instruments are unable to explain the variance in the predicted endogenous variables on the right (Bound, Jaeger, and Baker 1995).

Three tests were used to evaluate the IVs: the relevance of the instruments (Bound, Jaeger, and Baker 1995), overidentification tests, and the Durbin-Hausman-Wu test. The relevance test determines whether the instruments selected can explain the variation in the endogenous variable that is about to be instrumented. The test is an F-test on the joint significance of the instruments in each of the equations that predict income, household food availability, care, and health. The bias in the IV estimates in the nutrition equation will be approximated by (1/F)* (the bias from the OLS estimation). Hence, if F is 1, then these estimates are as biased as the OLS estimates.

The overidentification test determines whether the selected instruments belong in the second-stage equation itself. The test involves regressing the IV residuals from the nutrition equation on the left side and the instruments on the right side. The null hypothesis being tested posits that the instruments are uncorrelated with the error term from the nutrition equation and that the model is correctly specified. The test statistic is distributed as chi-squared, with the degrees of freedom equal to the number of instruments minus the number of endogenous variables on the right side.

The Durban-Hausman-Wu test determines whether the OLS and IV estimates differ significantly. To test for endogeneity, the actual and predicted values of food availability, care, and health, as well as income, are included in the second-stage equation for nutritional status. A joint test of significance is applied for the coefficients of the predicted variables. A rejection of the null hypothesis indicates that the IV estimates are significantly different from the OLS estimates.

Both OLS and IV results are presented so as to provide a range of estimates. For comparative purposes, each equation presents estimates from the structural and reduced forms. OLS is used to estimate the structural equations for food availability, health of the index child, care resources and practices, and nutritional status. There is no correction for any possible endogeneity of income in the first three equations or for income, calories, health, or care in the fourth equation. The IV method is used to estimate the structural equations using the predicted values of income, calories, health, and care that have been instrumented as a function of exogenous variables and a set of instruments to identify income, calories, care, and health.[55]

Finally, the estimates of the reduced-form equations for income, food availability, health of the index child, care resources and behaviors, and nutritional status are presented. These equations are functions of only the exogenous variables in each respective equation. To explore whether income has a direct effect on nutritional status (beyond its indirect effect through food availability, care, and health), nutritional status is estimated with and without income for both the OLS and IV estimation methods.

Determinants of Household Food Availability

Two different measures capture the quantity and quality of household food availability as the dependent variable. The first is total calories per adult equivalent unit (aeu) per day. The second measure, the price per 1,000 calories per aeu each day (kcal/aeu/day), captures the quality and economies of scale associated with household food availability. Household food availability is a function of food prices, expenditures, household demographics, and household tastes and preferences. Food price data were collected using market surveys at the community level, but a single-round survey over an eight-week period showed little temporal variation across markets in Accra. To account for any spatial variation, mean cluster prices for 16 enumeration areas are included for maize, cassava, yam, plantain, rice, wheat, tomato, and fish.

[55] Total per capita expenditure is used as a proxy for income. Household consumption expenditures are considered a more reliable indicator of permanent income than income itself, because they are less variable. Household expenditure data were easier to collect and tended to exhibit fewer measurement errors than income data.

Household composition is captured through linear indicators of the number of people in specified age and sex groups. To capture tastes and preferences related to basic household structure and differences in allocation priorities, the analysis includes a dummy variable for the sex of the head of the household—1 if the head is female, 0 if the head is male. The mother's age, education, and migration status are also included, since they may influence expenditure patterns and dietary preferences. The two dummy variables for population density at the community level are expected to capture any community-level effects that may influence household food availability. Each variable is equal to 1 if the community is classified as low density and 0 if it is high density (the reference variable is communities with medium density). The equations for food availability are

log of calories per aeu
or
price per 1,000 kcal/aeu/day = *g (predicted expenditures per log of aeu; household structure; sex of household head; mother's age, education, and migration status; prices for maize, cassava, yam, plantain, rice, wheat, tomato, and fish; and community density).*

The instruments for per capita expenditures are the age, education, and education squared of the head of the household; assets and assets squared; and home ownership. The age of the household head and assets are positive and significantly related to per capita expenditures. The OLS equation for predicting per capita expenditures is presented in Table 55.[56] The test results for the set of instruments used to predict per capita expenditures for food availability, health, and care are presented in each respective table. The instruments pass the relevance test and predict per capita expenditures well. The overidentification test in the food availability equation rejects the null hypothesis that the per capita expenditure instruments are uncorrelated with the error term and that the model is correctly specified. Similarly, the overidentification test rejects the null hypothesis for both the health equation and the care equation. For the Durbin-Hausman-Wu test, the OLS and IV estimates for household calorie availability are significantly different. For health and care, they are not.

The results of the calorie regressions using the log of household calories per aeu are presented in Table 56. As expected, per capita expenditure is positive and significantly related to household calorie availability. Increases in per capita income,

---

[56] Since 2SLS was used to estimate all equations, the log of per capita expenditure is predicted as a function of exogenous variables and instruments from the first stage (Table 55) and all the exogenous variables in the second stage (Table 57). Per capita expenditures were predicted in this same way for the equations for health, care, and nutritional status.

Table 55—Determinants of per capita expenditures

Variable	Variable name	Log of per capita expenditures	
		Coefficient	*t*-statistic
Education level of household head	edlevhh	–.005	0.331
Education level of household head^2	edlevhh2	.002	2.101*
Age of head of household	hhage	.004	2.099*
Household asset index	possess	.055	1.029
Household asset index^2	posses2	.029	2.120*
1 if house is owned	ownhouse	.028	0.618
Constant		13.38	113.07
Adjusted R^2		0.29	
F		38.6	
N		555	

* Significant at the .05 level.

proxied by per capita expenditures and with all other factors constant, are associated with higher household calorie availability. Household calorie availability decreases, however, with increases in the number of children between the ages of 5 and 14 and the number of young adult men between the ages of 15 and 34. In other words, households with relatively high numbers of school-aged children and men of prime working age have lower food availability. While children between the ages of 5 to 14 may eat less than adults, it is unlikely that young adult men have lower consumption needs, given their participation in wage labor and other income-generating activities.

Consistent with findings in the bivariate analysis, calorie availability is higher in female-headed households. Holding household structure constant, having a woman as head of household impacts calorie availability, reflecting differences in spending priorities between male- and female-headed households. The mean cluster price of cassava and tomatoes is significant and negatively correlated with food availability, while the mean cluster price of rice and red palm oil is positively associated with food availability.

The reduced form estimates are generally consistent with the structural equation estimates. Of the price estimates, only the price of tomatoes is significant and positive. Among the variables used as instruments for per capita income, only the age of the head of the household is significant. Households with older heads are associated with greater food availability.

In order to get an idea of the factors associated with food quality, the analysis determines the correlates of food prices per 1,000 kcal (Table 57). Relatively high levels of income and mother's education are significantly associated with more expensive diets. These results suggest that better-off and better-educated households choose a more expensive diet than households with less income and education, either by purchasing more expensive calories such as meat, fish, fruits, and vegetables or by purchasing more foods away from home. The findings in Chapter 5

Table 56—Determinants of household food availability (using household calorie availability)

Variable	Variable name	Log of household calorie availability per adult equivalent unit					
		Structural equation					
		OLS		IV[a]		Reduced form	
		Coefficient	*t*-statistic[b]	Coefficient	*t*-statistic	Coefficient	*t*-statistic
Maternal characteristics							
Mother's educational level	edlevpc	–.006	2.293*	–.003	0.826	.00003	0.007
Mother's age	ageyr_pc	.002	0.703	.003	1.245	.004	1.60
1 if mother is indigenous to Accra	migrpc1	–.016	0.402	–.012	0.288	–.022	0.428
1 if mother is migrant to Accra	migrpc2	–.006	0.165	.004	0.109	.021	0.502
Household characteristics							
Number of males 0–4 years	mal0_4	.059	2.097*	.040	1.318	.012	0.367
Number of males 5–14 years	mal5_14	–.043	2.541*	–.060	3.159*	–.092	4.514*
Number of males 15–34 years	mal15_34	–.064	2.906*	–.061	2.647*	–.070	2.598*
Number of males 35–49 years	mal35_49	–.029	0.699	–.015	0.348	–.041	0.782
Number of males over 50 years	mal50	.055	1.065	.034	0.624	–.070	0.973
Number of females 0–4 years	fem0_4	.076	2.682*	.045	1.431	–.005	0.146
Number of females 5–14 years	fem5_14	–.019	1.109	–.040	1.979*	–.075	3.649*
Number of females 15–34 years	fem15_34	–.025	1.887**	–.022	1.014	–.022	0.883
Number of females 35–49 years	fem35_49	.002	0.063	–.007	0.209	–.049	1.212
Number of females over 50 years	fem50	–.014	0.357	–.021	0.510	–.089	1.588
1 if female head of household	femhh	.156	3.754*	.133	2.99*	.141	2.595*
Log of per capita expenditures	lnpcexp	.415	15.948*	.268	3.852*	...	...

Instrument set for per capita expenditures							
Educational level of household head	edlevhh	...	...	...	...	.005	0.483
Educational level of household head^2	edlevhh2	...	...	...	...	–.0001	0.215
Age of household head	hhage	...	...	...	...	.005	2.062*
Assets	possess	...	...	...	...	.059	1.477
Assets^2	posses2	...	...	...	...	–.004	0.412
1 if own home	ownhouse	...	...	...	...	.027	0.667
Community-level variables							
Price of maize	maizepr	.0002	0.828	.0004	1.123	.0006	1.489
Price of cassava	cassavpr	–.001	2.637*	–.001	2.087*	–.0006	1.052
Price of yams	yampr	2.65e-06	0.004	.00004	0.509	.0001	1.520
Price of plantain	planpr	5.13e-06	0.056	.00004	0.412	.00005	0.406
Price of wheat	wheatpr	–9.97e-06	0.783	–.00002	1.132	–.00002	1.465
Price of rice	ricepr	.0003	2.156*	.0002	2.033*	.0003	1.847**
Price of tomatoes	tomatpr	–.0001	4.287*	–.00007	2.417*	–.00002	0.820
Price of red palm oil	oilpr	.0002	1.775**	.0001	1.492	.0001	1.303
Price of fish	fishpr	–.00002	0.820	–.00001	0.674	–.00001	0.484
1 if low density; 0 if medium	dense1	.071	1.015	.063	0.869	.082	0.949
1 if high density; 0 if medium	dense2	–.039	0.706	–.022	0.386	.020	0.300
Constant		1.91	3.621*	3.684	3.967*	6.61	12.395*
Adjusted R^2		0.38	0.342	0.342		0.09	
F		13.51		4.41		2.89	
N		552		550		552	
Relevance test (F-test)			15.12				
Overidentification test (chi^2)[c]			7.03*				
Hausman test (F-test)[d]			5.51*				

Notes: OLS is ordinary least squares; IV is instrumental variable.

[a] Log of per capita expenditures is instrumented.

[b] Absolute values of *t*-statistics are given.

[c] The test statistic is distributed as a chi^2, with degrees of freedom equal to the number of instruments minus one.

[d] The test statistic is distributed as an F-test with the degrees of freedom equal to (1, 510).

* Significant at the .05 level. ** Significant at the .10 level.

Table 57—Determinants of household food availability (using household calorie price)

Variable	Variable name	Log of price per 1,000 calories					
		Structural equation				Reduced form	
		OLS		IV[a]			
		Coefficient	*t*-statistic[b]	Coefficient	*t*-statistic	Coefficient	*t*-statistic
Maternal characteristics							
Mother's educational leveled	levpc	.005	2.381*	.004	1.751**	.007	2.514*
Mother's age	ageyr_pc	.007	0.424	.0003	0.165	.003	1.468
1 if mother is indigenous to Accra	migrpc1	.050	1.625	.048	1.574	.016	0.441
1 if mother is migrant to Accra	migrpc2	–.025	0.944	–.028	1.046	–.008	0.274
Household characteristics							
Number of males 0–4 years	mal0_4	–.048	2.227*	–.042	1.872**	–.031	0.993
Number of males 5–14 years	mal5_14	.004	0.334	.0084	0.599	.020	0.835
Number of males 15–34 years	mal15_34	–.0009	0.054	.0002	0.012	.025	1.037
Number of males 35–49 years	mal35_49	–.051	1.654**	–.050	1.583	.018	0.529
Number of males over 50 years	mal50	–.072	1.816**	–.062	1.517	–.054	1.026
Number of females 0–4 years	fem0_4	–.0008	0.039	.007	0.300	.005	0.147
Number of females 5–14 years	fem5_14	–.017	1.257	–.013	0.852	–.003	0.134
Number of females 15–34 years	fem15_34	–.001	0.081	–.003	0.172	.043	1.691**
Number of females 35–49 years	fem35_49	–.035	1.458	–.036	1.450	.018	0.529
Number of females over 50 years	fem50	–.061	1.983*	–.060	1.934**	–.012	0.260
1 if female household head	femhh	.002	0.081	.012	0.371	–.054	1.360
Log of per capita expenditures	lnpcexp	.265	13.333*	.302	5.816*	...	...

Variable	Name						
Instrument set for per capita expenditures							
Educational level of household head	edlevhh	...	...	...	...	–.008	1.062
Educational level of household head^2	edlevhh2	...	...	...	...	.0006	1.619
Age of household head	hhage	...	...	...	...	–.0009	0.549
Assets	possess	...	...	...	...	–.055	1.932**
Assets^2	posses2	...	...	...	...	.024	3.352*
1 if own home	ownhouse	...	...	...	...	064	2.203*
Community-level variables							
Price of maize	maizepr	.00001	0.048	–.0002	0.089.	.0002	0.971
Price of cassava	cassavpr	.0006	1.719**	.0005	1.518	.0009	2.240*
Price of yams	yampr	–.00003	0.670	–.00004	0.808	.00001	0.203
Price of plantain	planpr	.0001	2.709*	.0001	2.513*	.0002	3.104
Price of wheat	wheatpr	8.510	0.875	9.71e-06	0.979	7.670	0.699
Price of rice	ricepr	–.0001	1.509	–.0001	1.620	–.0001	1.054
Price of tomatoes	tomatpr	.00004	2.429*	.00004	1.699**	.00009	4.269*
Price of red palm oil	oilpr	–.0001	1.509	–.0001	2.070*	–.001	1.054
Price of fish	fishpr	.0003	1.851**	.00003	1.804**	.00004	2.317*
1 if low density; 0 if medium	dense1	–.074	1.376	–.0705	1.307	–.036	
1 if high density; 0 if medium	dense2	–.012	0.027	–.0180	0.416	.052	1.100
Constant		–.0001	1.509	–4.348	6.285*	–.65	1.702**
Adjusted R^2		0.45		0.45		.31	
F		17.78		12.42		8.70	
N		552		550		552	

Notes: OLS is ordinary least squares; IV is instrumental variable.

[a] Log of per capita expenditures is instrumented.

[b] Absolute values of *t*-statistics are given.

* Significant at the .05 level; ** Significant at the .10 level.

suggest that wealthier households do in fact select better-quality foods than low-income households. Although low-income households consume a larger percentage of more expensive street foods and meals purchased away from home, their calorie levels are lower. The mean price per 1,000 calories (regardless of the source) is also significantly lower for poor households.[57]

Determinants of Child Health

Child health status is measured using a visual analog scale (described in Chapter 6). Child health is a function of the environment (healthy or unhealthy) and of susceptibility and exposure to illness. Individual characteristics, such as age and sex, capture susceptibility to illness. Breast-feeding practices also capture susceptibility to illness, since children who are breast-fed exclusively for the first 4 to 6 months of their lives are exposed to fewer potentially pathogenic foods or liquids that can cause diarrhea. Exposure to pathogens can be captured as well by variables that affect children's immediate environment, such as contact with other children, the level of crowding in the household, the water source, sanitary conditions, and exposure to feces and to severe food contamination.

Other underlying determinants include maternal characteristics, household structure, and assets, measured by predicted expenditure (described in the previous section and in Table 56). Community-level variables are used to control for environmental sanitation, infrastructure, and the availability of health care. Because many of the variables are inputs into child health and reflect recent choices made by the household on use, they are endogenous to child health outcomes. These variables are not included in this version of the model.[58] The estimating structural equation for health is

Health visual analog scale squared/100 = *h (child's age, age squared, and sex; mother's age, education, education squared; sex of household head; predicted income; crowding; number of community toilets, hospitals, and clinics; and community density).*

[57] The log of household size was included in an alternative specification in the food availability equation when the log of price per calories was the dependent variable. Households with larger families are associated with cheaper diets, suggesting that economies of scale result from purchasing food in these households.

[58] Another version of the model was estimated including endogenous variables such as the water source used in the home, the type of toilet in the home, the presence of chicken feces in the compound, ownership of a refrigerator, the interaction between current breast-feeding and age group, and the interaction between measles immunization and age group. With a few exceptions, most of these variables are not significant. The interaction terms between breast-feeding and age are not significant for all age groups. However, the coefficients are positive for children who breast-fed between the ages of 0 and 12 months and negative for children who breast-fed from 13 to 17 months. Children who breast-fed in the older age group (over 18 months) have significantly poorer health outcomes. Children over the age of 9 months who have been immunized against measles have significantly higher health outcomes than children in that age group who have not been immunized.

Unfortunately, the results of the health equation, presented in Table 58, reveal little about the determinants of child health. Only a few coefficients are significant, indicating the difficulty of coming up with a set of regressors to explain child health status. Behrman and Deolalikar (1988) have noted the difficulty of finding strong associations, given the complex relationships between health outcomes and inputs. In the IV estimation, per capita expenditure is positively associated with better child health, and the result is significant. The age of the child and the age squared are significant and indicate that health improves as a child gets older.

Because of the poor results obtained using the visual analog health scale as the dependent variable, the same equation was estimated using probit on self-reported diarrhea in the past two weeks as an alternative dependent variable to capture child morbidity. The probit results are briefly discussed but not presented, because the estimates are not an improvement over those in Table 58. There is a negative and significant association between income and the child having had diarrhea once in the past two weeks. Age and age squared showed that older children are significantly more likely to get diarrhea. Children living in a compound household or in a community with one or more government hospitals had a higher probability of being sick with diarrhea.

The coefficients from the reduced form for child's health show a significant u-shaped relationship between maternal education and child health outcomes (Table 58, columns 5 and 6). Child health begins to improve only with a certain level of maternal education. The association between mothers' education and child health is positive when the mother has approximately eight years of schooling (middle school or junior high). In addition, a number of the demographic age and sex groups are significant, indicating a negative association between households with more children between the ages of 0 and 4 years and the health of the index child.

Lastly (and as the structural equation estimates also found), the health of the index child is significantly and negatively associated with the number of government hospitals in the community. The two communities in this sample that are closest to government hospitals have some of the poorest children's health outcomes in the sample. However, the economic status of the majority of households in the community, not the physical proximity to hospitals, explains the poor health status of children in these areas.

Determinants of Care

This model treats care somewhat differently than previous models. Previous studies have shown that maternal education is an important determinant of nutritional status (Behrman and Wolfe 1984). Typically, the pathway by which educational status affects nutritional status is not apparent in reduced form equations. The root of the difficulty lies in determining whether education improves nutrition through the effects of increased productivity (and thus earnings) or through improved caring practices (Sahn 1994). Some studies have tried to look at the impact of education on nutrition independent of increased productivity and earnings, but few studies try to include measures of care behaviors and practices (Strauss and Thomas 1995).

Table 58—Determinants of child's health (health visual analog for index child)

Variable	Variable name	Health visual analog scale (squared)					
		Structural equation				Reduced form	
		OLS		IV[a]			
		Coefficient	t-statistic[b]	Coefficient	t-statistic	Coefficient	t-statistic
Characteristics of child							
Age of child	agemo_ic	–1.134	2.703*	–1.076	2.515*	–1.132	2.664*
Age of child²	agemoic2	.025	2.287*	.024	2.084*	.026	2.296*
Sex of child	sex_ic	–.799	0.199	–1.796	0.434	–.773	0.196
Maternal characteristics							
Mother's educational level	edlevpc	–.615	0.939	–.709	1.056	–1.272	1.703**
Mother's educational level²	edlevpc2	.049	1.421	.04	1.103	.072	1.891**
Mother's age	ageyr_pc	–.188	1.127	–.266	1.506	–.191	1.125
Household characteristics							
Number of males 0–4 years	mal0_4	–3.030	1.118	–2.733	0.987	–2.931	1.092
Number of males 5–14 years	mal5_14	.990	0.750	1.862	1.303	.645	0.493
Number of males 15–34 years	mal15_34	–1.905	1.113	–2.303	1.316	–2.922	1.681**
Number of males 35–49 years	mal35_49	–1.469	0.462	–2.490	0.761	–2.413	0.716
Number of males over 50 years	mal50	3.954	0.987	4.754	1.129	2.955	0.634
Number of females 0–4 years	fem0_4	–2.008	0.759	–.471	0.164	–2.357	0.895
Number of females 5–14 years	fem5_14	.823	0.610	2.235	1.466	.864	0.646
Number of females 15–34 years	fem15_34	–.800	0.493	–.789	0.476	–.536	0.328
Number of females 35–49 years	fem35_49	–.656	0.265	.404	0.158	.750	0.286
Number of females over 50 years	fem50	.835	0.271	1.512	0.479	1.210	0.340
1 if female head of household	femhh	–4.106	1.258	–3.291	0.943	–2.288	0.650
Log of per capita expenditures	lnpcexp	3.218	1.554	12.915	2.259*	...	...
Number of people per room	crowding	2.545	1.064	–.593	0.198	3.032	1.294
1 if lives in compound house	cmpdhous	1.258	0.536	2.232	0.925	3.234	0.781

Instrument set for per capita expenditures							
Educational level of household head	edlevhh	. . .	. . .	. . .	. . .	.551	0.703
Educational level of household head^2	edlevhh2	. . .	. . .	. . .	. . .	−.011	0.282
Age of household head	hhage	. . .	. . .	. . .	. . .	.028	0.175
Assets	possess	. . .	. . .	. . .	. . .	3.558	1.369
Assets^2	posses2	. . .	. . .	. . .	. . .	−.471	0.709
1 if own home	ownhouse	. . .	. . .	. . .	. . .	−1.922	0.483
Community variables							
Number of public toilets	numtlts	1.490	1.272	1.717	1.436	1.571	1.342
Number of government hospitals	govthosp	−11.193	1.784**	−12.841	1.971*	−11.734	1.821**
Number of private hospitals	privhosp	1.237	0.464	−1.055	0.354	.278	0.102
Number of polyclinics	polyclin	−.591	0.216	−.156	0.056	−.349	0.127
Number of private clinics	privclin	.972	1.041	1.195	1.236	.708	0.075
1 if low density; 0 if medium	dense1	−11.788	1.788**	−9.763	1.422	−10.759	1.604
1 if high density; 0 if medium	dense2	−5.790	1.407	−6.912	1.639	−6.661	1.542
Constant		33.31	1.143	−94.734	1.239	73.124	6.464*
Adjusted R^2		0.060		.020		.0571	
F		2.23		2.26		2.03	
N		547		545		547	
Relevance test (F-test)				13.50			
Overidentification test (chi^2)[c]				2.17*			
Durbin-Hausman-Wu test (F-test)[d]				3.31			

[a] Log of per capita expenditures is instrumented.

[b] Absolute values of *t*-statistics are given.

[c] The test statistic is distributed as a chi-squared, with degrees of freedom equal to the number of instruments minus one.

[d] The test statistic is distributed as an F-test with the degrees of freedom equal to (1, 510).

* Significant at the .05 level. ** Significant at the .10 level.

Care resources include human resources, as measured by maternal characteristics; economic resources at the household level; and organizational resources at both the household and community levels (Chapter 7). Variables for maternal health, maternal age and education level, mother's ethnicity, household structure, predicted expenditure, and type of house capture the presence or absence of these resources. Mother's ethnicity is included as a proxy for cultural differences in maternal caring practices.[59] The dependent variable is the care index, standardized by the age of the child. The care index includes behaviors related to feeding practices and health-seeking practices (Chapter 7). The estimating equation for care is

Care index = *c (child's age, age squared, and sex; mother's age, education, ethnicity; sex of the head of the household; predicted income; living space, such as a single room; number of community toilets; community density).*

The age of the child is an important determinant of the type of care he or she receives. Among children under the age of three, the care index is lower for older children, indicating that caring behaviors and practices for preschoolers are suboptimal (Table 59).[60] The care resource that has a positive and significant impact on caring practices and behaviors is mother's education. There is no significant association between income and care, although the coefficient is positive. This result is consistent with the findings from Chapter 7 (Table 48), which identify lack of maternal schooling as the main constraint to child feeding practices. Breast-feeding practices were suboptimal across all households, however, regardless of socioeconomic status.

Type of housing is associated with care practices and behaviors. Care practices are negatively associated with households living in a single room compared with households in other types of living arrangements. Communities that have more public toilets are associated with better care practices and behaviors, although this outcome is significant only at the $p < 0.1$ levels. The reduced form estimates are in general agreement with the findings from the structural equations. Among the demographic variables, the estimates show that households with more males are associated with higher care indexes. In particular, the coefficients for males between the ages of 0 to 4 years, 15 to 34 years, and 35 to 49 years are positive and significant.

[59] Many of the variables that make up the care index also belong in the health equation. However, because of the problem of endogeneity of the care index in the health equation, variables reflecting care practices and resources are restricted to a select few, reflecting feeding practices, immunization, and hygiene.

[60] The care index used in the regression estimates differs slightly from the one described in Chapter 7, which is for children between the ages of 4 to 36 months. In order to keep as many index children in the sample as possible, the estimates use the care index for all children, including infants under the age of 4 months. Thus, the care index for children between 0 and 3.9 months is composed of two variables related to breast-feeding practices: whether the mother gave the child any food or liquid before initiating breast-feeding, and whether the mother is still breast-feeding the child.

Determinants of Nutritional Status

The primary relationship of interest here is the association between nutritional status and food availability, health, and care. Nutritional status is measured by the standardized height-for-age Z-scores. The effort to model the independent impact of the proximate determinants of child nutritional status amounts to an estimation of a structural equation for child nutrition. The estimating equation includes controls for the individual characteristics of the index child and the characteristics of both the primary caretaker and the household. A dummy variable captures the sex of the head of the household. The equation for nutritional status is

Height for age = *f (child's age, age squared, sex, and health; mother's education, age, and height; log of household size; sex of household head; log of food availability; and care index).*

Table 60 presents the coefficients for height-for-age Z-scores using IVs to control for the endogenous relationships among food availability, child health, and care (with and without income) and OLS (also with and without income). Table 61 presents the reduced form estimates, which provide a sense of the robustness of the parameter estimates on some exogenous variables. OLS estimates of height for age indicate that factors on the individual, maternal, and household levels are important determinants of nutritional status. Child nutritional status has a u-shaped relationship with the child's age, consistent with the descriptive statistics presented in Chapter 6. The sex of the child is not significantly related to nutritional status, indicating that there is no bias toward either male or female children. A mother's education and height are positive and significantly related to her child's height for age. The positive correlation between mother's height and child nutritional status is expected and has been noted in previous studies of malnutrition in Ghana (Alderman 1990) and elsewhere (Kennedy and Cogill 1987; Cebu Study Team 1992; Haughton and Haughton 1997). Food availability is positive but not significant, while care and health are positively and significantly associated with better nutritional status. When income is included, the coefficient on calorie availability becomes negative, but it remains insignificant. Income is positively associated with nutritional status, indicating that income might have other pathways to improved nutritional status outside of its effect on food, care, and health. Mother's education is not significant when controlling for income.

The IV estimation for height-for-age Z-scores includes predicted values for calories, care, and health. In stage one, calories, care, and health were regressed on all exogenous variables for the given input, all exogenous variables from the equation, and a set of instruments unique to each input. In the second stage, the predicted values for calories, health and care, and income were included in the regression. Table 62 lists the variables in the basic equation for estimating the nutritional status of the index child, along with the instrumenting equations for the other endogenous variables. Table 63 summarizes the relevance test, overidentification test, and

Table 59—Determinants of caring behaviors and practices (care index for index child)

Variable	Variable name	Care index					
		Structural equation				Reduced form	
		OLS		IV[a]			
		Coefficient	t-statistic[b]	Coefficient	t-statistic	Coefficient	t-statistic
Child characteristics							
Age of child	agemo_ic	–.147	4.892*	–.148	4.875	–.142	4.615
Age of child^2	agemoic2	.002	2.105*	.0017	2.105	.002	1.898**
Sex of child	sex_ic	–.315	1.086	–.351	1.188	–.312	1.071
Maternal characteristics							
Mother's educational level	edlevpc	.049	3.093*	.0394	2.086*	.034	1.906**
Mother's age	ageyr_pc	–.017	1.073	–.021	1.230	–.018	1.113
1 if mother is Gha/Adangbe	ethpc1	–.171	.638	–.178	0.659	–.251	0.866
1 if mother is Akan/Fanti/Ashante	ethpc2	–.435	1.579	–.457	1.633	.050	1.726**
1 if mother is Ewe	ethcp3	.146	.515	.1600	0.559	0.78	0.269
Household characteristics							
Number of males 0–4 years	mal0_4	–.290	1.492	–.267	1.346	–.277	1.414
Number of males 5–14 years	mal5_14	.010	.107	.048	0.442	.012	0.122
Number of males 15–34 years	mal15_34	–.186	1.419	–.190	1.432	–.224	1.682**
Number of males 35–49 years	mal35_49	–.322	1.387	–.340	1.444	–.452	1.784**
Number of males over 50 years	mal50	–.022	.075	.020	0.068	–.276	0.779
Number of females 0–4 years	fem0_4	.091	.482	.150	0.737	.068	0.356
Number of females 5–14 years	fem5_14	.122	1.239	.168	1.500	.139	1.409
Number of females 15–34 years	fem15_34	.007	.058	.005	0.045	–.004	0.034
Number of females 35–49 years	fem35_49	–.041	.222	–.008	0.043	–.138	0.699
Number of females over 50 years	fem50	.075	.310	.077	0.318	–.073	0.254
1 if female head of household	femhh	–.370	1.539	–.310	1.207	–.181	0.681
Log of per capita expenditures	lnpcexp	.025	.174	.335	0.851	...	...
1 if live in a single room	room	–.516	1.893**	–.399	1.292	–.502	1.806**

Instrument set for per capita expenditures							
Educational level of household head	edlevhh	...	...	...	...	.063	1.175
Educational level of household head^2	edlevhh2	...	...	...	...	–.002	0.627
Age of household head	hhage	...	...	...	...	.016	1.348
Assets	possess	...	...	...	...	.204	1.085
Assets^2	posses2	...	...	...	...	–.046	0.0950
1 if own home	ownhouse	...	...	...	...	–.019	0.102
Community variables							
Number of public toilets	numtlts	.125	1.659**	.130	1.707**	.128	1.691**
1 if low density; 0 if medium	dense1	–.063	.184	–.010	0.029	–.057	0.164
1 if high density; 0 if medium	dense2	.176	.800	.172	0.775	.116	0.521
Constant		.32	.150	–3.894	5.412	–.178	0.185
Adjusted R^2		.23		0.220		0.225	
F		7.34		7.24		6.16	
N		517		515		516	
Relevance test (F-test)				14.97			
Overidentification test (chi^2)[c]				4.53*			
Durbin-Hausman-Wu test (F-test)[d]				0.56			

Notes: OLS is ordinary least squares; IV is instrumental variables.

[a] Log of per capita expenditures is instrumented.

[b] Absolute values of *t*-statistics are given.

[c] The test statistic is distributed as a chi^2, with degrees of freedom equal to the number of instruments minus one.

[d] The test statistic is distributed as an F-test with the degrees of freedom equal to (1,510).

* Significant at .05 level. ** Significant at .10 level.

Table 60—Determinants of child's nutritional status (stunting): Structural equations

		Structural equations for height-for-age Z-score							
		OLS 1		OLS2		IV 1[a]		IV 2[a]	
Variable	Variable name	Coefficient	*t*-statistic[b]	Coefficient	*t*-statistic	Coefficient	*t*-statistic	Coefficient	*t*-statistic
Proximate determinants									
Household food availability	lncalaeu	.074	0.614	–.127	0.901	.440	1.071	–.153	0.320
Care index	careidx3	.053	1.930**	0.054	1.955*	–.098	0.958	–.029	0.284
Health of index child	icvas_sq	.006	2.993*	.005	2.604*	.012	1.830**	.001	0.188
Child characteristics									
Age	agemo_ic	–.064	3.424*	–.067	5.565*	–.080	3.368*	–.082	3.587*
Age^2	agemoic2	.001	2.248*	.001	2.346*	.001	2.263*	.001	2.574*
Sex	sex_ic	.090	0.971	.096	1.043	.091	0.937	.097	1.027
Maternal characteristics									
Educational level	edlevpc	.016	1.768**	.009	0.769	.018	1.742**	.003	0.252
Age	ageyr_pc	.004	0.463	.003	0.388.	–.002	0.204	–.001	0.142
Height	ht_pc	.054	6.720*	.055	6.868*	.054	6.249*	.057	6.689*
Household characteristics									
1 if female head	femhh	.018	0.175	.106	1.011	–.003	0.027	.156	1.251
Size	lnhhsize	.033	0.271	.099	0.800	.122	0.778	.199	1.280
Log of per capita expenditures	lnpcexp	...	...	0.267	2.667*	...	...	.515	2.273*
Constant		–9.97	6.364*	–12.17	6.942*	–13.35	4.031*	–15.53	4.651*
Adjusted R^2		0.18		0.19		0.10		0.16	
Overidentification test[c]					26.80*		31.77*		
Durbin-Hausman-Wu test[d]					1.20		1.50		

Notes:

[a] Per capita expenditures, household food availability, health analog scale, and care index are instrumented. The first-stage OLS estimates for food, care, and health are not presented but are estimated as endogenous based on the equations and instruments presented.

[b] Absolute values of *t*-statistics are given.

[c] The test statistic is distributed as a chi^2, with degrees of freedom equal to the number of instruments minus three.

[d] The test statistic is distributed as an F-test with the degrees of freedom equal to (3,510).

* Significant at .05 level. ** Significant at .10 level.

Durbin-Hausman Wu test for the height-for-age Z-score regression using IVs. The relevance test for food availability, health, and care indicates that these instruments do not predict their respective endogenous variables very well. Because the F-tests are greater than one, the IV estimates are likely to be less biased than the OLS results, but the F-values are not large enough to validate the instrument set. The over-identification test for the nutrition equation suggests that the instruments do not perform well, in that they are correlated with the nutrition error term. The Durbin-Hausman-Wu test cannot reject the null hypothesis that the IVs and OLS are identical.

These results indicate that the instruments for food availability, care, and health are not powerful and do not explain enough of the variations in the first-stage dependent variables for proper identification. (The exception is the set of instruments for income.) Given the high number of potentially endogenous variables in the height-for-age equation, it was difficult to find appropriate instruments that were correlated with the one endogenous variable but not the others. Thus, it is not surprising that in the second-stage equation, the set of instruments are correlated with the error term, and the IV and OLS are not significantly different from one another. Given that the instruments in the equation are weak, OLS estimates are just as good as IV estimates until better instruments can be identified.

In the IV estimates, neither food nor care is significantly associated with nutritional status. The weak relationship between household food consumption and nutrition in cross-sectional analysis has been noted in a number of economic studies (Alderman 1989; Alderman 1990; Haddad et al. 1996). Household food availability is a poor proxy for individual food intake, since it does not take intrahousehold distribution into account.

Given that this study models the intake of very young children (from 0 to 3 years of age), it is not unusual that the association between household-level food availability and nutritional status is insignificant. Typically, children in this age group derive a large proportion of their energy from breast milk. For instance, in developing countries children age 1–2 obtain, on average, more than half their daily calories from breast milk (WHO 1998). In this sample, 55 percent of the index children were still breast-feeding, suggesting that breast milk was providing much of their dietary energy intake. Complementary foods contributed a relatively small number of calories. The difference between malnourished and well-nourished children, then, is the result not of extra calories from complementary foods but of factors such as the quality of these foods, the number of overall feedings per day, and other maternal feeding choices.

The care index loses significance in both the IV estimates, with and without income, while long-term child nutritional status (measured by height-for-age Z-scores) is positively associated with better health. From the IV estimates, it appears that health is the factor that most affects child nutritional status—but with several important caveats. First, the visual analog scale is both highly subjective and correlated with nutritional status, reflecting a combination of poor growth and high morbidity from the mother's perspective. Therefore, many of the variables that are

Table 61—Determinants of child's nutritional status (stunting): Reduced form estimates

Variable	Variable name	Reduced form for HAZ			
		OLS 1		OLS 2	
		Coefficient	*t*-statistic[b]	Coefficient	*t*-statistic
Child characteristics					
Age	agemo_ic	–.080	4.208*	–.080	4.259*
Age^2	agemoic2	.001	2.735*	.001	2.807*
Sex	sex_ic	.140	0.776	.117	1.242
Maternal characteristics					
Educational level	edlevpc	–.028	0.036	–.015	0.441
Education level^2	edlevpc2	.001	0.659	.001	0.767
Age	ageyr_pc	–.001	0.114	–.0006	0.078
Height	ht_pc	.046	5.558*	.047	5.742*
Household characteristics					
1 if female head	femhh	.146	0.912	.124	0.977
Size	lnhhsize	...	...	–.048	0.341
Number of males 0–4 years	mal0_4	–.098	0.809	...	...
Number of males 5–14 years	mal5_14	–.038	0.635	...	...
Number of males 15–34 years	mal15_34	.049	0.620	...	...
Number of males 35–49 years	mal35_49	–.050	0.329	...	...
Number of males over 50 years	mal50	–.334	1.583	...	...
Number of females 0–4 years	fem0_4	–.123	1.027	...	...
Number of females 5–14 years	fem5_14	.005	0.084	...	...
Number of females 15–34 years	fem15_34	–.035	0.470	...	...
Number of females 35–49 years	fem35_49	.067	0.563	...	...
Number of females over 50 years	fem50	–.199	1.215	...	...
Community-level variables					
1 if low density; 0 if medium	dense1	.449	0.884	...	...
1 if high density; 0 if medium	dense2	–.021	0.067	...	...
Instrument set					
Food availability					
1 if mother is indigenous to Accra	migrpc1	–.079	0.331	–.040	0.169
1 if mother is migrant to Accra	migrpc2	.062	0.495	.081	0.657
Price of maize	maizepr	–.002	0.578	–.0003	0.241
Price of cassava	cassavpr	–.001	0.295	–.003	0.965
Price of yams	yampr	–.001	0.877	–.0006	0.802
Price of plantain	planpr	.001	0.585	.0004	0.383
Price of wheat	wheatpr	–.000	0.489	–4.39e-06	0.054
Price of rice	ricepr	–.001	0.657	–.0003	0.291
Price of tomatoes	tomatpr	.000	0.565	.00003	0.177
Price of red palm oil	oilpr	–.000	0.203	.0003	0.743
Price of fish	fishpr	.000	1.143	.0002	1.311
Care					
1 if mother is Gha/Adangbe	ethpc1	.321	1.194	.263	1.000
1 if mother is Akan/Fanti/Ashante	ethpc2	.222	1.112	.212	1.076
1 if mother is Ewe	ethpc3	.220	1.097	.197	1.009
1 if live in single room	room	–.103	0.560	–.070	0.384

(continued)

Table 61—Continued

Variable	Variable name	Reduced form for HAZ			
		OLS 1		OLS 2	
		Coefficient	*t*-statistic[b]	Coefficient	*t*-statistic
Health					
Number of people per room	crowding	–.134	1.188	–.111	0.990
1 if lives in compound house	cmpdhous	–.044	0.221	.011	0.057
Number of public toilets	numtlts	–.174	0.730	–.036	0.307
Number of private hospitals	privhosp	–.365	0.477	–.065	0.139
Number of polyclinics	polyclin	.118	0.601	.045	0.277
Number of private clinics	privclin	–.308	0.952	–.133	0.896
Per capita expenditures					
Educational level of household head	edlevhh	–.006	0.182	–.012	0.350
Educational level of household head^2	edlevhh2	.001	0.659	.001	0.842
Age of household head	hhage	.008	1.180	.001	0.208
Assets	possess	–.002	0.015	.031	0.267
Assets^2	posses2	.015	0.480	.009	0.285
1 if own home	ownhouse	.034	0.166	–.052	0.270
Constant		–3.98	0.626	–7.365	2.742
Adjusted R^2		0.15		0.15	
F-test on all variables		3.00		3.71	
N			549		549

Notes: HAZ is height-for-age Z-score; OLS is ordinary last squares.
[a] Absolute values of *t*-statistics are given.
* Significant at the .05 level. ** Significant at the .10 level.

correlated with the health outcomes are also correlated with nutritional status. This relationship makes finding a set of regressors that are correlated to nutritional status but not to health particularly difficult. Ideally, however, health outcomes and nutritional status should be modeled simultaneously.

Second, based on the conceptual model (Figure 2), the health concept should be represented by a variable that captures a healthy environment and access to health services. The visual analog scale is highly correlated with nutritional status and is difficult to predict, given the difficulty in finding a valid set of instruments. For this reason, it does not pick up the effects on nutritional status of a healthy environment and access to health services.

A final cause for concern is the questionable validity of the instruments used to predict health, care, and food. A set of instruments that is relatively weakly correlated with the endogenous variable that needs instrumenting can seriously bias the estimates, even if only a weak relationship exists between the instruments and the error term in the structural equation (Bound, Jaeger, and Baker 1995). The reduced form estimates presented in Table 61 show that when the instruments for income, food, health, and care are included directly in the height-for-age equation as exogenous

Table 62—Variables used to estimate nutritional status of index child and instrumenting equations

Variable	Variable name Dep. var =>	Basic equation: Nutritional status of index child (HAZ)	Instrumenting equations for other endogenous variables: Per capita expenditures (lnpcexp)	Food availability (lncalaeu)	Health of index child (icvas_sq)	Care of index child (careidx3)
Age of child	agemo_ic	✓	✓	✓	✓	✓
Age of child^2	agemoic2	✓	✓	✓	✓	✓
Sex of child	sex_ic	✓	✓	✓	✓	✓
Predicted health of index child	icvas_sq	✓				
Predicted care index	careidx3	✓				
Age of primary caregiver	ageyr_pc	✓	✓	✓	✓	✓
Caregiver's educational level	edlevpc	✓	✓	✓	✓	✓
Caregiver's educational level^2	edlevpc2	✓			✓	
Maternal height	ht_pc			✓	✓	✓
Log of household size	lnhhsize	✓	✓			
1 if female head of household	femhh	✓	✓	✓	✓	✓
Predicted per capita household expenditures	lnpcexp	✓		✓	✓	✓
Predicted household calorie availability per adult equivalent unit	lncalaeu	✓				
Number of males 0–4 years	mal0_4			✓	✓	✓
Number of males 5–14 years	mal5_14			✓	✓	✓
Number of males 15–34 years	mal15_34			✓	✓	✓
Number of males 35–49 years	mal35_49			✓	✓	✓
Number of males 50 and over	mal50			✓	✓	✓
Number of females 0–4 years	fem0_4			✓	✓	✓
Number of females 15–34 years	fem15_34			✓	✓	✓
Number of females 35–49 years	fem35_49			✓	✓	✓
Number of females 50 years and over	fem50			✓	✓	✓

1 if low density; 0 if medium	dense1		✓	✓	✓
1 if high density; 0 if medium	dense2		✓	✓	✓
Educational level of household head	edlevhh	✓	✓	✓	✓
Educational level of household head^2	edlevhh2	✓	✓	✓	✓
Age of household head	hhage	✓	✓	✓	✓
1 if house is owned	ownhouse	✓	✓	✓	✓
Household asset index	posses1	✓	✓	✓	✓
Household asset index^2	posses2	✓	✓	✓	✓
Price of maize (cedis/kilogram)	maizepr		✓		
Price of cassava (cedis/kilogram)	cassavpr		✓		
Price of yams (cedis/kilogram)	yampr		✓		
Price of plantain (cedis/kilogram)	planpr		✓		
Price of wheat (cedis/kilogram)	wheatpr		✓		
Price of rice (cedis/kilogram)	ricepr		✓		
Price of tomatoes (cedis/kilogram)	tomatpr		✓		
Price of red palm oil (cedis/kilogram)	oilpr		✓		
Price of fish (cedis/kilogram)	fishpr		✓		
1 if PCIC is indigenous to Accra	migrpc1		✓		
1 if PCIC is migrant to Accra	migrpc2			✓	
1 if government hospital in community	govthosp			✓	
1 if private hospital in community	privhosp			✓	
1 if polyclinic in community	polyclin			✓	
1 if private clinic in community	privclin			✓	
Number of people per room	crowding				✓
1 if household lives in a room	room				✓
1 if Gha/Adangbe	ethpc1				✓
1 if Akan/Fanti/Ashanti	ethpc2				✓
1 if Ewe	ethpc3				✓

Note: HAZ is height-for-age Z-score.

Table 63—Results from relevance test, overidentification test, and Durbin-Hausman-Wu test for household calorie availability, health visual analog, care index, and standardized height-for-age of index child, IV regression analysis

Dependent variable	Relevance test for income instruments (F-test)	Relevance test of instruments for standardized height for age of index child (HAZ) (F-test)	Overidentification test (Chi^2)	Durbin Hausman-Wu test (F-test)	Implication
Per capita total household expenditure	n.a.	6.67	n.a.	n.a.	Instruments are good predictors in first stage.
Household calorie availability	15.12	1.41	7.03 (reject null)	5.51 (reject null)	Instruments are good predictors in first stage; instruments are correlated with error in second stage; IV and OLS are different in second-stage equation. Look for improved instruments until overidentification test null is not rejected.
Health visual analog of index child	13.50	1.79	2.17 (reject null)	3.31 (fail to reject null)	Instruments are good predictors in first stage; instruments are correlated with the error in second stage; IV and OLS are not different in second-stage equation; Look for improved instruments until overidentification test null is not rejected.
Care index for index child	14.97	1.9	4.53 (reject null)	0.56 (fail to reject null)	Instruments are good predictors in first stage; instruments are correlated with the error in second stage; IV and OLS are not different in second-stage equation. Look for improved instruments until overidentification test null is not rejected.
Standardized height for age of index child	n.a.	n.a.	26.80 and 31.77 31.77	1.2 and 1.50 (fail to reject null)	Instruments are weak. Use OLS unless better instruments can be identified.

Notes: OLS is ordinary least squares; IV is instrumental variables; n.a. is not applicable.

variables, most of the coefficients for the explanatory variables are insignificant.[61] The poor predictive power of these covariates may be a result of multicollinearity, model misspecification, or omitted variables.[62]

Maternal characteristics, such as mother's height and education, are positively and significantly correlated to child's height for age. A mother's education is mediated through care practices and behaviors and child health and also has a direct effect on child nutritional status. Better-educated women are able to combine inputs to care and health to improve children's nutritional status. When predicted income is included, the coefficient on the health variable drops and becomes marginally significant. Income is positive and significant. The coefficient on food availability turns negative and remains insignificant. Once income is included, the coefficient on mother's education drops slightly and becomes insignificant, shedding some light on the additional effects of maternal education on nutritional status (primarily through employment opportunities and income-earning potential).[63]

A Participatory Analysis of Child Malnutrition

To assess perceptions of child malnutrition, researchers conducted participatory concept-mapping exercises with groups of women in different areas of the city.[64] The concept map in Figure 10 was made by a group of working mothers in a peri-urban community, most of whom have little or no formal education. This concept map, like many similar ones made by various groups throughout the city, reveals a strong perception of the link between malnutrition and poor health, but other factors highlighted in the map include most of the variables that come out of the multivariate analysis. Poor care and feeding practices are noted as a cause of malnutrition. Poor sanitation and environmental hygiene are noted as factors leading to illness.

---

[61] A number of alternative specifications were tried to improve the instruments for food availability, health, and care. Among these was the inclusion of a set of enumeration area dummy variables to capture enumeration area effects. However, when these were included in the models for food availability, health, and care, they were highly correlated with other community-level variables, leading to multicollinearity and suggesting that the community variables may already be picking up these fixed effects.

[62] These results suggest the need to identify new variables that measure a healthy environment and access to health services and to find better instruments for predicting health, care, and food availability, especially when collecting a single round of survey data.

[63] For a detailed analysis focusing on the relationship between care practices and child nutritional status, see Ruel et al. (1998). Using a subsample of this data set for children age 4–36 months, the researchers show that good care practices could compensate for low maternal education and insufficient income. The study finds that household income is not a statistically significant determinant of child nutritional status when maternal schooling and caring practices are included in the model. Thus, household income affects child nutritional status only through maternal schooling and caring practices. In the current study, when income is included in the model, the income effect exceeds the effect of maternal schooling. These differences are most likely caused by differences in the samples and in definitions of maternal schooling and income.

[64] The exercises consisted of asking participants in focus groups to brainstorm all possible causes of child malnutrition, then noting each response on a card and asking participants to arrange the cards in a way that reflected their understanding of causes and effects. For complete methodological details, see Maxwell et al. (1997).

Figure 10—A participatory analysis of the causes of child malnutrition

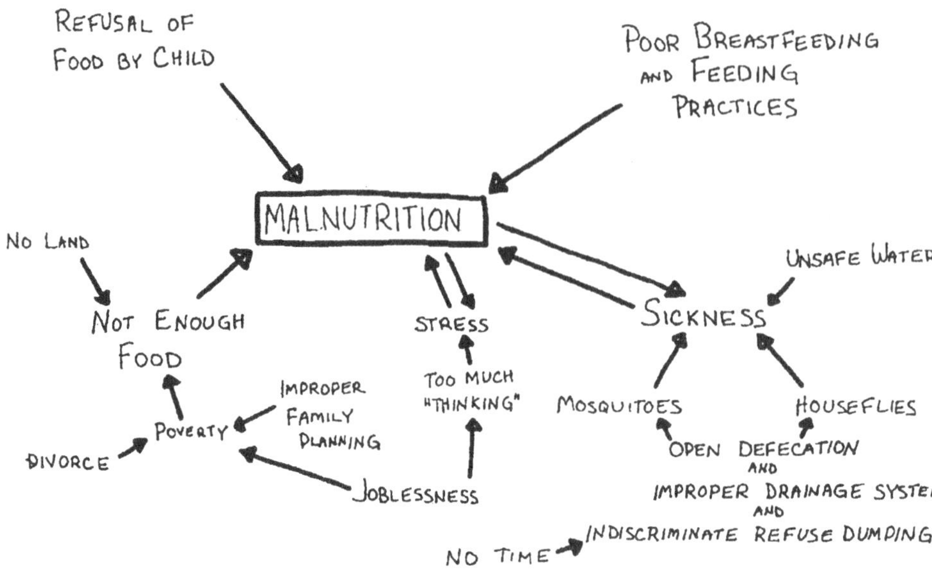

Note: This diagram was constructed by a working women's group during the study.

Food insecurity is seen as a result of joblessness, landlessness,[65] and several features of household structure. Stress (in this case, stress on the mother due to financial worries) is seen as contributing to child malnutrition. The appetite of the child is viewed as an independent factor. These factors are simply listed and organized according to their perceived relationship to malnutrition. They are not weighted or ranked in terms of importance.

These maps give important information in several areas. First, they show that some of the coping activities people use are unavoidable. Ignorance of the consequences of these strategies is not the reason for some of the less "successful" coping strategies—it is rather a lack of alternatives. These maps clearly indicate that mothers are aware of consequences of, for example, poor feeding practices and poor environmental hygiene, but time and income constraints may not permit alternative actions. This fact tends to support the notion that maternal education affects child nutritional status through improved earning capacity.

Second, these maps provide the locus for a discussion of useful interventions at the community and household levels, because the maps identify commonly perceived problems and leverage points and underscore the findings of the multivariate analysis. For example, this study and others note the difficulty of ferreting out the rela-

[65] This particular concept map came from a peri-urban community where agricultural land was rapidly being lost, and many members of the community had previously been farmers.

tionship between household food availability and nutritional status using cross-sectional data. Yet maternal perceptions of the link between food insecurity and child malnutrition, and of the causes of food insecurity, are quite strong across all the groups that constructed these maps. This participatory analysis indicates that programs aimed at enhancing mothers' ability to earn an income or to improve environmental sanitation and reduce illness would be broadly acceptable as interventions whose real aim is to improve child nutrition. Clearly, maternal perceptions of the causes of child malnutrition complement the quantitative findings.

What the Findings Show

Both the OLS and IVs indicate that the strongest determinants of child nutritional status are the individual characteristics of the child and mother. Household food availability is not a significant determinant of the child's nutritional status, while the OLS estimates indicate that care and health are important inputs. However, individual energy intake, which is not measured here, may still be an important determinant of child's nutritional status.

The findings from the multivariate analysis support many of the associations described in previous chapters. As expected, higher incomes do lead to increased household food availability, higher-quality diets, and better health for the child, but not to significantly improved care practices and behaviors. These findings are consistent with the bivariate analysis in Chapter 7, which shows that good care practices are not associated with any socioeconomic factors, including income. Rather, maternal schooling is strongly associated with good care practices and positive behaviors. Mother's education matters. Maternal schooling is associated with higher levels of household food availability, higher-quality diets, better care practices and behaviors, and better nutritional outcomes.

CHAPTER 10

Urban Livelihood Security: Assets, Vulnerability, Trade-offs, and Coping

The challenge posed by the conceptual framework for livelihood security is to understand the ways people organize their assets, capabilities, and activities—and their means of coping—to gain access to their basic requirements. Some of the major pieces to this puzzle, described by Davies (1996) as "sources of entitlement," were discussed in Chapter 4: household structure and organization, labor and income-generating activities, and coping and reciprocal exchange. Others, described as "calls on entitlement," were analyzed in Chapters 5 and 7: resource allocation, particularly patterns of expenditure; food consumption and acquisition of other basic needs; and care. Still others—health and nutritional status—are outcomes, at least in the short term, but in the long term they are also necessary inputs to the ability to work and to cognitive ability. These chapters have also identified the major determinants of and constraints to the primary outcomes of interest—income, food availability, health, care, and nutritional status.

This chapter addresses several issues suggested by the analyses in foregoing chapters. First, it examines the trade-offs people have to make to survive in the city, given the constraints on people's ability to earn sufficient income and the cost of acquiring even basic needs in an urban environment. Second, it seeks to determine what the patterns of coping suggested by these trade-offs say about the range of choices available. In other words, it asks whether people's coping strategies are "successful." And third, it identifies those groups that are the most vulnerable in the city.

Trade-offs and Coping: Are Coping Strategies Successful?

At least three major categories of trade-offs emerge from the analysis in Chapters 3 to 7. These include the trade-off between consumption and savings (or investment); the trade-off between food and other basic necessities; and perhaps most important, the trade-off between maternal work and child care. People's choices in each of these categories have important implications for all the outcomes of interest in this study.

Consumption versus Savings

The analysis in Table 33 reveals a small but notable group of households (39 in all, or about 7 percent of the sample), mostly headed by male migrants, that are sending large amounts of money out of the city (or, in a few cases, to other households within the city). None of the other expenditure categories are particularly unusual for this group. The senders are clearly sacrificing food consumption in the short run in order to be able to send these remittances and thus fall into the "questionable" category noted in Chapter 5. The remittances amounted to a mean of about $150 in the previous year, with some as high as $1,000. The households are fairly evenly distributed across per capita expenditure quintiles but have a higher-than-average number of income-generating activities (2.3). None of them had sought assistance from another household in the form of a transfer of money or goods.[66] This group is clearly unique. Other net remitting households, for the most part, do not fall into this "questionable" food security category. But indeed there is nothing "questionable" about this particular subgroup—its priorities are clear.

For the *kayayoo*—the migrant female market porters who come to Accra mostly from northern Ghana in order to earn money and save for marriage—the major trade-off is also between consumption and savings (Agarwal 1994). To save money, they often live in squalid conditions, and many of them have small children. Because of the children, they are a visibly vulnerable group, although one with clear objectives. Their stay in the city is usually limited. One young woman summarized the objectives of this group. She stated that she minimized all housing and consumption expenditures and used most of her money to buy the cloth, bowls, and cooking pots she needed for marriage. She added, "I am seriously saving to buy a sewing machine and to get some capital, so when I go back home I can trade with it."

Food Consumption versus Other Basic Needs

Table 33 shows the proportion of households in the city with adequate levels of calorie availability but relatively high shares of food expenditures in the overall budget. This group is considered vulnerable because a small price or income shock could quickly undermine their consumption status. Table 34 shows that over half of all female-headed households in the city fall into this category, as do a high proportion of the predominantly female occupational groups—especially petty traders and street food vendors.

In conventional analysis of food security, the "food secure" and the "vulnerable" groups would be classified together (because they have adequate calorie availability),

[66] Unfortunately, the questionnaire did not include a question asking how long respondents intended to stay in the city, so it is not possible to speculate on whether this use of money amounts to urban-based investment in rural areas or is simply a coping strategy based on urban-rural kinship linkages.

Table 64—Characteristics of food security groups: Income-generating activities, dependency ratio, transfers and budget shares, per capita expenditure, and coping ability

Variable	Group			
	Food secure	Vulnerable	Questionable	Food insecure
Number	115	219	93	132
Mean dependency ratio[a]	1.01	1.23	1.16	1.44
Income-generating activities per household	1.87	1.77	2.06	1.90
Proportion of income from transfers (percent)	19.1	25.0	14.7	17.0
Food share of total budget	27.9	65.3	37.1	62.9
Health share of total budget[a]	6.7	3.4	6.4	3.3
Education share of total budget[a]	1.3	1.5	2.4	2.0
Street food share of food budget (percent)[a]	28.5	29.9	32.5	41.1
Per capita expenditure (₵1,000)[a]	1,933	930	916	503
Child forced to drop out of school (percent)[a]	5.2	8.3	7.5	11.0

[a] Significant difference among groups ($p < 0.05$).

and the "questionable" and the "food insecure" groups would be classified together (because they do not).

Table 64 compares the four food security groups identified in Table 33 for dependency ratio and several income and expenditure measures.[67] The mean number of income-generating activities at the household level does not differ significantly across these groups. Dependency ratios are higher for the "vulnerable" and "food insecure" groups. Households in the "vulnerable" group make a clear trade-off between food consumption and other basic needs. Both health and education receive a significantly lower share of the household budget in this group, reflecting some of the sacrifices that are made to achieve relatively adequate food consumption.

Budget shares for health in "food secure" and "questionable" households are considerably higher and food shares considerably lower than in the "food insecure" or "vulnerable" groups.[68] The "vulnerable" group receives the highest proportion of income from transfers. The "food insecure" group has by far the lowest income

[67] In a conventional analysis of food security, the "food secure" and "vulnerable" groups would be grouped together (because they have adequate calorie availability), as would the "questionable" and the "food insecure" groups (because they do not).

[68] Food budget shares were used to construct these groups. The comparison is made only to show the contrast with budget shares for nonfood basic necessities.

levels and clearly just cuts all costs to get something to eat, even if it is not enough. An unemployed man in a densely populated neighborhood put the situation of these city dwellers this way: "At the end of the day, if you can at least eat something, you can survive, but we can't manage all these other things." (The "other things" included school fees, medical expenses, and child support.)

Case studies provide abundant evidence of the way in which nonfood costs are cut. People often minimize health care costs by diagnosing illnesses at home and treating them with cheap drugs instead of going to a clinic. The diagnosis is considerably more expensive than the drugs, at least in the case of common illnesses such as malaria, so many people seek a diagnosis only if they cannot successfully treat themselves (or their children). Seeking treatment from an herbalist is another strategy, although it is not necessarily associated with cost-cutting.

Examples of ways to cut food expenditures have already been noted (see Chapter 5). In the case studies, people most often mentioned the "divisibility" of street foods as a cost-cutting strategy, that is, they consume smaller portions of prepared food when money is scarce, rather than buying a quantity of ingredients to prepare the dish themselves. Survey respondents said they most often made changes to their diets when they needed to cut food costs, usually by eating less or buying less expensive foods. The "vulnerable" group relies on coping strategies that increase the short-term availability of food, including borrowing food or money, purchasing on credit, or relying on a transfer from someone outside the household. This group is also the one that is most likely to seek out transfers in time of need. The "vulnerable" group apparently achieves adequate food consumption in the short term, but it is vulnerable to income shocks and health care crises (also in the short term). This increases long-term vulnerability by relying on coping strategies that increase indebtedness and by failing to invest in education.

However, the results in Table 65 suggest that the strategy works, at least to some extent. Children in the "vulnerable" category have a higher mean height for age than children in the "food insecure" group, and the proportion of stunted children is smaller in this group. But the health status of both mothers and children in this category is no different from the health status of mothers and children in other

Table 65—Food security groups: Outcomes

Groups	Health of primary caregiver of index child	Index child health	Mean height-for-age Z-Score[a]	Percent stunted[a]
Food secure	54.9	59.6	–0.68	11.4
Vulnerable	55.4	53.4	–0.87	13.7
Questionable	52.3	53.8	–0.77	15.1
Food insecure	55.1	53.7	–1.08	22.7

[a] Significant difference ($p < 0.05$.)

groups, despite the fact that health expenditures seem to be sacrificed for food. This strategy may therefore be an example of successful coping.[69]

The "food insecure" group's coping strategies tend to be oriented toward rationing or getting by with the little that is already available. Although households seek out assistance, they do so less frequently. School children in this group tend to drop out of school at high rates, suggesting that these households sacrifice long-term investments in education for short-term survival. Reliance on street foods is a particularly important strategy for the food insecure group, with the share of street foods in the household food budget at over 40 percent of the total. But as noted in Chapter 5, on a per calorie basis, street foods are among the most expensive foods. Relying on such foods, then, is an example of a coping strategy that is not successful. The group most dependent on street foods is the one that can least afford to be spending its limited money on more expensive calories.

Table 65 compares these groups in terms of outcomes. Despite the fact that households in the "vulnerable" category spend significantly less on health care, mothers and children in these households do not seem to suffer because of it: there are no differences in health outcomes among all these groups. Figures are not shown for other measures of health, such as the frequency of diarrhea, fever, or other symptoms in the index child, because they do not reveal any significant differences. Differences among groups show up more clearly for nutritional status. The prevalence of stunting among the "food secure" group (11.4 percent) is half that of the "food insecure" group (22.7 percent), though the mean per capita expenditure is four times higher in the "food secure" group. These results are consistent with the multivariate analysis presented in Chapter 9, which shows no significant relationship between household food availability and height-for-age Z-scores.

Maternal Work versus Care

The third important trade-off is between maternal employment and childcare. Maternal work is negatively related to nutritional status, and the relationship is clearly confounded by the age of the child.[70] The age of the child—or, more precisely, the time that has elapsed since birth—is clearly one factor in determining when the mother goes back to work. Case study and focus group evidence strongly suggests that two primary factors determine when mothers return to their income-generating activities: first, how "rested" the mother feels, and second, the imperative of earning an income. Focus group discussions on this issue made clear that mothers know

[69] It is impossible to determine whether relying on transfers as a coping strategy is "successful" or not, because these data give little information about the reciprocal obligation. Focus group participants tended to say they preferred income that they had earned themselves to transfer income, because then they were free of such obligations. But such obligations are not an indication of coping "failure."

[70] The results of the multivariate analysis in Chapter 8 confirm the positive relationship of care to nutritional status, but the relationship between maternal work and care (explored in Chapter 7) is less clear.

Table 66—Characteristics of working and nonworking primary caregivers of index child

Age group of index child	Working primary caregiver: Number	Time working	Receives assistance from father	Proportion of income from transfers	Nonworking primary caregiver: Number	Receives assistance from father	Proportion of income from transfers
		(hours/day)	(percent)			(percent)	
0–12 months	91 (45.7)	4.47	87	9.6	105 (52.8)	85	26.6
12–24 months	147 (72.8)	6.50	73	21.5	50 (24.8)	86	38.9
24–39 months	120 (77.4)	7.15	73	8.7	32 (20.0)	59	36.7

Note: Numbers in parentheses are the share of the total sample.

[a] Unemployed group not shown. Only three caregivers in the 0–1 year age group were unemployed only five in the 1–2 year age group, and just three in the 2–3 age group.

they often return to work at a time when their children are most vulnerable—and that their return to work increases that vulnerability. On average, women return to work anywhere from 3 to 18 months after birth.[71] At about this age, children are often old enough to be mobile and have to be tended constantly. But that fact does not remove the imperative of earning an income. One market vendor with a child about a year old put the dilemma in stark terms: "When I have to leave my child [to go back to work] my stomach burns me,[72] but I have to work to earn money. Caring for your child is important, but you also have to earn money to provide for your child."

Because both the health and nutritional status of children appear to be worst in the 1–2 age group, the entire sample was broken into three groups according to the age of the index child (Table 66).[73] Mean per capita expenditure at the household level does not differ among the groups. Total per capita expenditure among households with children age 1–2 is significantly higher (by 260,000) if the mother works. This factor alone speaks volumes about why women have to return to work. Per capita expenditure also differs by sex of the household head. Male-headed households have much higher per capita expenditure, a finding already noted in Chapter 4.

A variety of maternal and household-level factors were compared across these groups (Table 66). Receiving financial assistance from the child's father (without

[71] The survey results reveal that after giving birth women take off a mean period of 18 weeks (just over 4 months). But this figure does not take into account women who had stopped working when they gave birth and had not yet returned to work by the time of their interview, so 18 weeks is likely to be a low estimate.

[72] Literal translation of a Ga colloquialism.

[73] 0–12 months; 12.01–24 months; and older than 24.01 months.

regard to marital status) is another important factor in the trade-off between work and care. The proportion of households reporting that they receive such assistance drops from 87 percent in the first year to 73 percent in the second year for mothers who go back to work. The figure remains the same for nonworking mothers, however. The proportion of income from transfers is higher in the group with index children between 1 and 2 than it is for the group with children between 0 and 1—a somewhat unexpected result. However, the proportions and actual amounts of transfer income are lower for households with working mothers than for households with nonworking mothers. Given that the data are cross-sectional, identifying the cause and effect relationship here is impossible. Either mothers go back to work because they are getting less help from fathers and less transfer income, or help from fathers and transfer income are lower because the mother is working (and presumed to be more self-sufficient). Findings from women's focus groups strongly suggest the former.

Many factors affect the trade-off between work, care, and nutritional status, including the place of work, the amount of time spent at work, and alternate sources of income, including assistance from the father of the child. But at root, the imperative of earning a livelihood is the deciding factor in whether and when a mother returns to work. One working mother with a year-old child summarized the situation: "If you are wealthy, or your husband is taking good care of you, you can even stay [off work] for three years. But things are now hard. I *have* to earn an income."

Leverage Points for Intervention

Constraints to livelihood security tend to fall into several categories: those related to household structure and assets, those related to income-generating activities, and those related to the trade-offs just discussed. Some of these constraints suggest leverage points for intervention—either policy or programmatic. These are explored further in Chapter 11. Constraints related to household structure revolve primarily around the availability of labor. Households with relatively limited labor resources or a high dependency ratio tend to have both low incomes and poor food security and health and nutrition outcomes. Likewise, female-headed households (which tend to have fewer labor resources and higher dependency ratios) have relatively low incomes and poor nutritional outcomes, although their spending priorities may protect food security. Given these constraints, leverage points for either policy or program interventions are limited, with a few exceptions, particularly interventions that increased labor productivity, especially those mentioned below.

Constraints related to income-generating activities revolve around education and skills, access to credit, the regulatory framework for work (especially informal work), the availability of alternative forms of childcare, and the level of organization among independent microentrepreneurs. These constraints affect several groups in particular: working mothers, the unemployed, unskilled laborers, petty traders, and street food vendors. Farmers in peri-urban areas are constrained by a separate set of factors—mainly rapid urban sprawl, environmental degradation, and land laws regarding the loss of usufruct rights. These groups are among the most vulnerable identified during the study. With the exception of peri-urban farmers, many of them overlap to a large degree with the groups identified with household structure constraints—for example, female-headed households where the main occupational activity is petty trading and selling street foods. This set of constraints does lend itself to intervention by either policy or programmatic means, or both, however. Education, skill training, credit for small enterprises, and creation of an enabling environment for small-scale trade are some examples.

The trade-offs discussed in this chapter also suggest leverage points for intervention. In terms of income generation, the strategy many mothers use—allocating time to work rather than to childcare—is clearly successful. In terms of child welfare outcomes, however, it is not. But the trade-off is not straightforward: the relationship hinges not only on the mother's work status, but on her workplace, the amount of financial assistance she receives from the father or from other sources, the availability of alternative childcare, and on the child's age. Most working mothers do not feel they have any choice in the matter: the imperative to earn an income is paramount. Without it, these women would be even less able to care for their children. This outcome has implications for women's employment (and self-employment) and for the provision of alternative childcare.

This analysis has shown that people deal with constraints to livelihoods in different ways. Yet nearly every outcome analyzed here and many of the determinants of these outcomes are related to poverty, income, employment, and the ability to earn a living. The links among poverty, food insecurity, and malnutrition are complex in the urban context, yet these relationships underpin much of urban life. This fact was underlined during one of the early community studies. After attempting to respond to the many questions posed about work, food security, care, and nutrition, one woman simply threw up her hands and said "shika, shika, shika!" ("[The answer to all your questions is] money, money, money!").

Clearly, the issues raised here can be addressed in many ways that do not rely solely on "money, money, money." Policy-related interventions, for example, could help create an environment that enables improved self-employment practices in the city, without the injection of major amounts of money. But resources will be required, both to operate programs and interventions and, given the findings about the dispersed and "hidden" nature of urban poverty, food insecurity, and malnutrition, to successfully identify deserving participants in those programs. The final chapter of this report makes recommendations and suggests priorities for policies and programs.

CHAPTER 11

Conclusions and Policy Recommendations

The study sought to understand the nature of poverty, vulnerability, and food insecurity in an urban setting, using both qualitative and quantitative research methods. The preceding chapters have discussed the study's methodology and presented its findings. This concluding chapter addresses several questions presented by the foregoing analysis. In the context of increasing urban poverty, who are particularly vulnerable groups? What are the main sources of vulnerability? And, building on the analysis in Chapter 9 and the leverage points noted in Chapter 10, what can be done to reduce vulnerability? These questions are applied to both policy and program interventions by the state, local government or municipality, and civil society organizations[74] active in the urban context. The appendix builds on the analysis in Chapter 8 to create the indicators that are needed for effective targeting, monitoring, and evaluation of the interventions suggested here.

Vulnerable Groups in Urban Settings

Previous research identified several groups that had been particularly hard hit by the economic changes that took place in Ghana during the 1980s and 1990s. The qualitative research that preceded this study confirmed these findings. Four groups in particular are considered to be highly vulnerable. The first group consists of low-income urban wage earners, who were hurt not only by the economic crisis but also by the reforms undertaken to counter it. Members of this group have seen their wage income drop and their ability to earn a living through secondary self-employment constrained by high inflation, lack of access to credit, and a sometimes hostile regulatory environment (Ga Mashie Study Team 1996; Bortei-Doku Aryeetey and Aryeetey 1996; Gayi 1995).

[74] Civil society organizations include nongovernmental organizations (NGOs), community-based organizations, and the entire range of informal local organizations.

The second group is the city's indigenous Ga population. This group has been identified as vulnerable in part because of the loss of traditional livelihoods (fishing and farming), which are becoming increasingly difficult to maintain as the city expands into formerly rural areas (Ngleshie-Amanfro Study Team 1996; Bortei-Doku Aryeetey and Aryeetey 1996).[75] The "new" urban poor make up the third group. This group emerged in the aftermath of the economic reforms and includes those recently "redeployed" (involuntarily retired or laid off) from the civil service (Gayi 1995; Alderman, Canagarajah, and Younger 1994). The final group comprises households headed by single women. This group is particularly vulnerable in terms of income, which tends to be low. It is also at serious risk in case of illness or injury to the primary income earner, since such households are likely to have few wage earners (Bortei-Doku Aryeetey and Aryeetey 1996).

The results of the income analysis presented in this study confirm the vulnerability of these groups, with one exception. The number of households in the sample that included a person redeployed within the past five years was very small—only 26 households in the sample, or less than 5 percent of the total. The status of this group cannot be adequately assessed with such a small number.[76]

This study has also suggested a number of other groups that must be considered vulnerable. These include female-headed households; households with few assets, particularly labor; working women with children in the 0–2 age groups; and women with low educational levels. Households in all these groups are vulnerable largely because they have so few assets, particularly human assets—that is, labor, education, and salable skills. For some groups, vulnerability is defined by the ability to earn a livelihood (or, in the case of the unemployed, by the inability to do so). These categories include farmers in the peri-urban areas of the city, where land is rapidly disappearing to nonagricultural uses; petty traders, particularly those in the central business district who are subject to harassment by city authorities; street food vendors; and unskilled laborers.[77]

Vulnerability for still other livelihood groups revolves around the issues of poor employment opportunities, lack of access to credit, and a regulatory environment that constrains the activities of the urban self-employed. One special group derived from the analysis of household food security includes those who consume an adequate amount of food but spend a disproportionate part of their total income to acquire it. For this group, vulnerability is clearly the result of a low income combined with the trade-offs that accompany coping strategies. Several other categories not

[75] Vulnerability is not simply a matter of ethnicity or place of birth, however. The indigenous population of Accra is evenly divided among all income groups (Table 60), yet the old indigenous communities are the locus of some of the worst poverty in the city. A complex combination of factors leads to this group's vulnerability.

[76] This small number is almost certainly the result of the survey's sampling strategy, which focused on households that included a child under the age of three. The redeployment exercise has been running since the mid-1980s, and many of those redeployed were middle-aged civil servants who were unlikely to have small children.

[77] Farmers in the peri-urban area constitute a special group, because their vulnerability revolves around the loss of usufruct land rights and the rapid expansion of the city.

particularly identified by the survey but noted during qualitative fieldwork or by other researchers include street children (Apt van Ham, Blavo, and Opoku 1991), and at least one other occupational group—the *kayayoo* or young migrant, female market porters (Agarwal 1994).

Clearly, if an individual or household falls into more than one of these categories, vulnerability increases. For example, a low-income female-headed indigenous household in which the mother has to take a small child with her to work in the market is extremely vulnerable. Such combinations are unfortunately not uncommon in Accra.

Policy Interventions to Reduce Urban Vulnerability

Two preconditions must be met before governments, donor agencies, and others can begin addressing vulnerability and poverty in urban areas. Results of interviews and workshops with policymakers in Accra suggest that these preconditions may be more important than the policy initiatives themselves. The first precondition is simply accepting that rapid urban growth is a fact of life in Sub-Saharan Africa. Neither agriculture-led growth policies nor industrial decentralization policies have been successful in reversing the trend in urban growth, particularly of primary cities (Becker, Jamer, and Morrison 1994). The temptation to promote accelerated rural development to stem the tide of urban drift—and therefore the growth of urban poverty—remains strong. But the results of this study and others (OECD 1995) suggest that urban problems cannot be dealt with by addressing rural issues.

The second precondition is recognizing that urban poverty exists. When this study began in 1996, poverty in Ghana was considered a predominantly rural problem. National governments must recognize that because of the rapid pace of urban population growth and the increase in urban poverty, the problems this study has identified are likely to intensify over time—both in Accra and in many other cities in Sub-Saharan Africa. While urban areas are on average better off than rural areas, results of this and other studies show that cities are outpacing rural areas in population growth and that poverty, food insecurity, and malnutrition are increasing more rapidly. While rural-urban indicators of poverty may change only slowly, recognizing the long-term trend is the first step in addressing this problem. Achieving a balance between rural and urban poverty alleviation initiatives is imperative.

For the foreseeable future, interventions aimed at reducing poverty through traditional measures such as food or cash transfers may be severely limited by budgetary constraints. Therefore, interventions may need to incorporate indirect means of alleviating poverty, such as improving the capacity of the urban poor to earn a living. Designing these interventions requires an understanding of what is unique about urban livelihoods. This study has highlighted many singularities, including reliance on cash incomes, dependence on purchased foods, the importance of labor and marketable skills as assets, and social relations among urban groups, among many others.

Interventions at the National Level

To reduce overall poverty, a major national policy strategy must link urban growth and other economic issues. With adequate planning, urban population growth—which increases demand for many goods and services—can be a powerful force for spurring growth in agricultural production. The results of this study indicate, for instance, that urban diets differ significantly from traditional rural diets. Urban consumption patterns have begun to favor predominantly imported rather than domestically grown staple foods. Some of the changes in consumption patterns are the result of tastes and preferences associated with higher incomes. However, these patterns are also emerging among low-income households. As demands on women's time increase, women are turning to time-saving foods that are relatively easy to prepare and cook.

To address this issue, Ghana needs to continue researching and developing processed foods derived from domestically produced foodstuffs—maize, yams, plantains, and cassava. Such foods are important if domestic food production is to meet the majority of the country's food needs in years to come. Similarly, domestic rice production, processing, and marketing must be expanded, and the quality of domestic rice will need to improve in order to compete with imports. This study did not investigate the policy trade-offs in national food security between increased domestic food production and exports plus increased food imports. This policy issue must be addressed in light of the changes in urban dietary preferences noted here.

A second national poverty reduction strategy suggested by this study addresses the needs of a range of vulnerable groups—female-headed households, working mothers and their children, and households short on labor. The study strongly indicates that for these groups, higher female educational levels are positively related both to increases in income and to improved child health and nutritional status. (The latter relationship holds even after controlling for the effect of household income.) The implications of this result are clear: education for girls and women is a very good investment because it reduces poverty in the future. Efforts to increase women's educational levels can be accompanied by focused, relevant educational messages on childcare and child welfare—in particular, messages related to the importance of breast-feeding. These should include information about the importance of breast-feeding exclusively for a minimum of four months (and six if possible), avoiding prelacteal feedings, and not using water as a substitute for breast milk. These educational messages need to be targeted to the health sector in general, not just to individual mothers.

Policy Interventions at the City and Local Level

A special category of vulnerable groups in this study includes farmers and other inhabitants of peri-urban areas. In greater Accra, this group is composed largely but not exclusively of indigenous people. The city's rapid, uncontrolled expansion has resulted in landlessness, the loss of traditional livelihoods, and the creation of a new class of urban poor from a group that was previously reasonably secure. Specific policy initiatives to address the problems these groups face include a land-use policy for peri-urban areas; an environmental policy with enforcement capacity for quarrying, sand mining, and land reclamation; and compensation for displaced agricultural workers.

Virtually all the sprawl in Accra that leads to the rapid loss of farmland is caused by the construction of single-family dwellings on individual plots. Tax incentives for low-cost, high-rise housing can slow this loss. For ecological and social reasons, some peri-urban land should be zoned for agricultural or greenbelt use in perpetuity. The construction boom in the city and the demand for building materials are destroying large swathes of peri-urban land, because the mining of sand and even topsoil is driven by an insatiable demand for construction and landscaping materials. The sand contractors rarely reclaim mined land, which is useless if it is not reclaimed. The peri-urban districts on their own are not able to control the practice, so the need for a firm national policy on licensing and land reclamation—with strong enforcement mechanisms—is urgent. When land will inevitably be lost to agriculture because more space is required for urbanized land uses, farmers need to be compensated for the loss of their livelihood. Current laws allow for compensation for family land but make no provision for other categories of land or for nonindigenous people.[78] Compensation need not be in the form of cash. Other possibilities include retraining that will allow displaced farmers to enter other occupations and access to credit and technology that will allow them to stay in agriculture, but on a more commercial, intensified basis.

For other groups described above, the major forms of vulnerability revolve around poor employment opportunities, lack of access to credit, and the regulatory environment for self-employment. Both local government and civil society organizations have roles to play in addressing these issues. For local governments, employment and enhanced possibilities for self-employment are the first priorities for social policy. Employment policies must take into account the attempts of low-income urban residents to diversify their incomes, gain access to credit, and work in a regulatory environment where they are taxed at a fair rate and are free from harassment by authorities.

The policy initiatives that will do most to enhance the potential for self-employment are in the regulatory sphere. Here again, certain preconditions apply. First, local governments must recognize the right of all Accra's citizens to earn a living, including in the informal economy. Historically, the municipal administration in Accra (as in most other large African cities) has tended to view the informal economy as a problem to be solved rather than as a resource for dealing with the employment problem. As a result, many informal entrepreneurs with few other ways

[78] Family land is a special category of land tenure in the peri-urban area.

to earn a living have been subjected to considerable harassment by municipal authorities.

One of the major areas of contention is street vending. The streets are the best place for hawkers and vendors to sell their wares, but Accra's city authorities blame them for congestion in the central business district (see Chapter 4).[79] The central business district, however, offers plentiful customers, relatively high prices, and rapid turnover. Traders must choose between a confrontation with the authorities there or trading in their home neighborhood, where customers are fewer, turnover is slower, and profit margins are therefore lower. The trade-off between profits and relative safety is one many traders are not willing to make. The government's approach to the problem—building new markets away from the city center (see Chapter 4)—has thus far not been successful, since vendors are reluctant to move.

Several other possibilities for easing constraints on petty traders are available, however. One is to set aside certain areas of the central business district for pedestrians and petty traders only—a possibility already under discussion. A second is strengthening the capacity of nascent traders' associations and working directly with their leaders. This approach would give political voice to the concerns of small-scale entrepreneurs and help develop self-regulatory mechanisms for informal trade activities. However, to date attempts to develop or strengthen such associations have come almost exclusively from the top, and in some quarters the associations are viewed as the municipal administration in disguise.

Street foods are another source of regulatory concern. The metropolitan authorities view street foods primarily as a source of food contamination and therefore as a threat to public health. But the issue of street foods is much more complex: street foods are also an important source of food for consumption, a key coping strategy, and a livelihood for a large number of women in Accra. The city cannot regulate the hygenic conditions of all street food vendors, as the number of vendors is too large. Further, there is no clear evidence that street foods should be singled out as a public health threat. Given the conditions under which some street foods are prepared, sold, and consumed, however, the authorities certainly have cause for concern. Local area associations of street food vendors that can self-inspect and regulate hygienic conditions would be good for business and for public health, but forming such associations will require the municipal authorities to take a different approach—one that emphasizes participation and collaboration rather than control.

Promoting this type of approach requires a central body or roundtable where all parties can meet. In such a forum, policy issues can be raised, initiatives debated, and decisions taken openly and transparently with the participation of all stakeholders. This body should include not only the district assemblies but also occupational and consumer groups, organizations of civil society, and other interested parties. While the local government has the final say over the regulatory environment,

---

79 The municipal police have other motives for harassing traders, including the extraction of petty payments.

civil society organizations can complement government efforts to reduce poverty, primarily through programs that provide training, credit, assistance with managing microbusinesses, and alternative forms of childcare for working women. These organizations also have an important role to play in advocating changes in the regulatory environment and in the fundamental attitudes necessary to ensure the success of policy initiatives.

A final important component of poverty reduction in cities is the question of safety nets. This study did not directly address the issue of formal safety nets, although it did examine the informal safety net an enabling environment for self-employment would provide. However, important changes in other types of informal safety nets—particularly interhousehold transfers—have implications for planners of formal safety nets. And given the relatively low level of spatial clustering in human welfare outcomes in the city (including income, food security, health and nutritional status of children, and child mortality), any approach to safety nets should be based on a household or occupational targeting approach, not geographic targeting. This point has major implications for programming. Low-income areas will still be a priority. But mechanisms are needed to identify the truly vulnerable wherever they live and work in the urban area. Such targeting and monitoring systems can be very simple. This study developed a set of indicators that can be used to develop both targeting and monitoring mechanisms (see the Appendix).

Accra, like many other cities in the West African region, is growing at a rapid pace and is experiencing a rapid increase in poverty levels and deterioration in indicators of nutritional status. Trends in poverty and malnutrition show that the problems identified by this study are likely to intensify over the coming two decades—conclusions broadly echoed by the West Africa Long-Term Perspectives Study (OECD 1995). These same trends can be observed in many cities, but the results of this study indicate that governments and civil society organizations can act to reduce poverty in cities and to mitigate the worst impacts of rapid urbanization on the vulnerable. Demographic trends alone will increasingly shift the locus of these problems into urban areas over the next 20 years. The time to begin to deal with the problems of urban livelihoods, poverty, food insecurity, poor health, and malnutrition is now.

APPENDIX

Indicators of Urban Vulnerability and Food and Nutrition Insecurity

This study used several categories of indicators that summarize a variety of factors related to outcomes and that can be used to identify vulnerable groups. Creating some of these indicators require expensive and time-consuming survey methodology. But a number of proxy indicators were developed for this study that require less time and expense. These indicators can help in identifying vulnerable groups for targeting purposes and in monitoring the impact of interventions on such groups. They fall into several general categories: demographic, livelihood, income and expenditure, food security, and health and nutrition. They are briefly described here, but more complete descriptions can be found in Accra Study Team (1998) and in the various citations mentioned below.

Demographic Indicators

The major demographic indicators used here are household headship, age structure and the dependency ratio, available labor in the household, and education. These indicators all define significant factors in household vulnerability. For the most part, however, there is no simpler way to acquire the necessary information about these characteristics than by using the standard survey methodology described in Chapter 2 and in Annex 1 of Accra Study Team (1998). For targeting purposes, however, the indicators are simple to use. For instance, monitoring who is dropping out of school and for what reasons is a good way to identify households in crisis, if monitoring can be done at the local primary school level.

Livelihood Indicators

The main outcome measure for livelihood security is income, which for the purposes of this study was taken as reported expenditure. Other indicators include assets (human, financial, physical, and social), measures of income diversification, the primary income-generating activity of the head of household, and maternal work status and place of work. At a more aggregated level, the level of unemployment and the ratio of workers in the formal and informal sectors of the urban economy were taken as indicators. Total per capita expenditure was the main proxy measure of income at the household level. (Gathering this information is time-consuming and expensive and thus is not useful for targeting or program monitoring purposes).

A simple index of housing environment and consumer durable possessions was also developed for this study (Accra Study Team 1998). This index is similar to the asset indexes used in many other studies. It worked reasonably well and is relatively easy to duplicate. Not only does it directly capture the issue of assets, it correlates reasonably well with per capita income (r = 0.514) and can distinguish expenditure groups. Qualitative measures, particularly livelihood profiles, present an alternative indicator. As noted in Chapter 4, however, in this study they sometimes gave results that differed from the surveys.

Food, Security, Health, and Care

The traditional food security indicator of caloric availability outlined in Chapter 5 requires an enormous amount of time and expense to construct, and it is further complicated if combined with food budget shares. This study experimented with an alternative measure of household food security that is based on the frequency and severity of coping strategies. It worked reasonably well, particularly for ruling out cases—that is, for identifying households in vulnerable groups that are not food insecure. This method is described in great detail in Maxwell et al. (1999).

A complete child and maternal health recall was beyond the means even of this study, so only some information on recent episodes of illness was collected. However, the study experimented with the health visual analog scale described in Chapter 6. In the absence of a complete morbidity recall, determining the accuracy of this very quick and inexpensive method for estimating longer-term health status is impossible. However, it correlates well with expected determinants of health, categories of care, and health-seeking behaviors and is significantly related to nutritional status. Further trials of this method in other urban studies of care and nutrition are planned. The indicators of care are complex to compile, but on the whole, maternal education was the best predictor of children's care status.

Nutritional Status

There are no good measures of nutritional status other than child and maternal anthropometry—particularly child height for age. Although collecting the data involves extensive training and field supervision, the information is easy to compile and process. Maternal body mass index (BMI) is not a good indicator of child nutritional status and especially not of household food security outcomes. However, weight-for-age Z-scores are a reasonable proxy for height-for-age Z-scores (r = 0.736; R^2 = 0.541) when the score is the sole variable used to predict height for age.

This point is important, for two reasons. First, measuring the weight of young children does not require the same high degree of staff training and supervision as measuring height or length. Second, the maternal and child health mobile clinics in the city are already screening on the basis of weight for age, so some systems are already in place.

References

Accra Study Team. 1998. Promoting urban food and nutrition security for the vulnerable in the greater Accra metropolitan area. Technical report to the World Health Organization. International Food Policy Research Institute, Washington, D.C., and Noguchi Memorial Institute for Medical Research, Legon, Ghana. Photocopy.

Acquah, I. 1958. *Accra survey: A social survey of the capital of Ghana (Gold Coast), 1953–1956.* Accra: University of Ghana Press.

Aforo, A. 1997. Report of the miniconsultation on street trading and hawking in Accra. Accra Sustainable Programme, Accra. Photocopy.

Agarwal, S. 1994. Bearing the weight: The Kayayoo—Ghana's working girl child. United Nations Children's Fund, Accra. Photocopy.

Akpedonu, P. 1996. Persistent diarrhea in Ghana. Progress report to Japan International Cooperation Agency. Noguchi Memorial Institute for Medical Research, Legon, Ghana. Photocopy.

———. 1998. Progress report: Food contamination study. Noguchi Memorial Institute for Medical Research, Legon, Ghana.

Alderman, H. 1989. New research on poverty and malnutrition: What are the implications for research and policy? Paper presented at the World Bank–International Food Policy Research Institute Conference on Poverty, Airlie House, October 25–28. World Bank, Washington, D.C.

———. 1990. *Nutritional status in Ghana and its determinants.* Policy Analysis Working Paper 3. Washington, D.C.: World Bank.

———. 1994. Ghana: Adjustment's star pupil? In *Adjusting to policy failure in African economies,* ed. D. Sahn. Ithaca, N.Y., U.S.A.: Cornell University Press.

Alderman, H., and M. Garcia. 1993. *Poverty, household food security, and nutrition in rural Pakistan.* Research Report 96. Washington, D.C.: International Food Policy Research Institute.

Alderman, H., and P. Higgins. 1992. *Food and nutritional adequacy in Ghana.* Working Paper 27. Washington, D.C.: Cornell Food and Nutrition Policy Program.

Alderman, H., and G. Shively. 1996. Economic reform and food prices: Evidence from markets in Ghana. *World Development* 24 (3): 521–534.

Alderman, H., S. Canagarajah, and S. Younger. 1994. Consequences of permanent layoff from the civil service: Results from a survey of retrenched workers in Ghana. In *Rehabilitating government: Pay and employment reform in Africa,* ed. D. Lindauer and B. Nunberg. Washington, D.C.: World Bank.

Amis, P. 1995. Making sense of urban poverty. *Environment and Urbanization* 7 (1): 145–157.

Amis, P., and C. Rakodi. 1994. Urban poverty: Issues for research and policy. *Journal of International Development* 6 (5): 627–634.

Apt van Ham, N., E. Q. Blavo, and S. K. Opoku. 1991. Street children in Accra: A survey report. Department of Sociology Report, University of Ghana, Legon. Photocopy.

Armar, M. A. 1989. Maternal energy status, lactational capacity and infant growth in rural Ghana: A study of the interactions of cultural and biological factors. Ph.D. dissertation. University of London.

Armar-Klemesu, M. 1996. Nutrition and persistent diarrhoea in childhood: A study of interactions and outcomes. Progress Report to the Japan International Cooperation Agency. Noguchi Memorial Institute for Medical Research, Legon, Ghana. Photocopy.

Armar-Klemesu, M., and D. Maxwell. 1998. Urban agriculture in the Greater Accra Metropolitan Area. Technical report to the International Development Research Centre. Noguchi Memorial Institute for Medical Research, Legon, Ghana.

Asenso-Okyere, W. K., F. A. Asante, and M. Nubé. 1997. Understanding the health and nutritional status of children in Ghana. *Agricultural Economics* 17 (1): 59–74.

Atkinson, S. 1992. Food for the cities: Urban nutrition policy in developing countries. Urban Health Program, Health Policy Unit. Department of Public Health and Policy, London School of Hygiene and Tropical Medicine, London.

Atkinson, S. 1995. Approaches and actors in urban food security in developing countries. *Habitat International* 19 (2): 151–163.

Austin, J. E., et al.1976. *Urban malnutrition—Problem assessment and intervention guidelines.* Washington, D.C.: World Bank.

Baah-Nuakoh, A. 1996. Enhancing the role of the informal sector in the Ghanaian economy. *FASS Bulletin: Faculty of Social Studies* 1 (1): 1–17.

Baker, J., and P. Ove Pedersen. 1992. *The rural-urban interface in Africa.* Uppsala: The Scandinavian Institute of African Studies.

Barker, D. J. P. 1994. *Mothers, babies, and disease in later life.* London: British Medical Journal Publishing Group.

Bates, R. 1981. *Markets and states in tropical Africa.* Berkeley, Calif., U.S.A.: University of California Press.

Beaton, G. H. 1983. Energy in human nutrition: Perspectives and problems. *Nutrition Review* 41 (11): 325–340.

———. 1993. Which age group should be targeted for supplementary feeding? In *Nutritional issues in foreign aid.* ACC/SCN Symposium Report Nutrition Policy Discussion Paper No. 12. Geneva: ACC/SCN.

Becker, C., A. Jamer, and A. Morrison. 1994. *Beyond urban bias in Africa.* Portsmouth, N.H., U.S.A.: Heinemann.

Behrman, J. R., and A. B. Deolalikar. 1988. Health and nutrition. In *Handbook of development economics,* vol. 1, ed. H. Chenery and T. N. Srinivasan. Amsterdam: Elsevier.

Behrman, J., and B. L. Wolfe. 1984. More evidence on nutrition demand. *Journal of Development Economics* 14 (1–2): 105–128.

———. 1997. How does mother's schooling affect the family's health, nutrition, medical care usage and household sanitation? *Journal of Econometrics* 36: 185–204.

Benneh, G., J. Songsore, J. Nabila, A. T. Amuzu, K. A. Tutu, Y. Yangyuoru, and G. McGranahan. 1993. *Environmental problems and the urban household in the Greater Accra Metropolitan Area, Ghana.* Stockholm: Stockholm Environment Institute.

Bennett S., T. Woods, W. M. Liyanage, and D. L. Smith. 1991. A simplified general method for cluster-sample surveys of health in developing countries. *World Health Statistics Quarterly* 44 (1): 98–106.

Bentley, M. E., M. M. Black, and E. Hurtado. 1995. Child-feeding and appetite: What can programmes do? *Food and Nutrition Bulletin* 16 (4): 340–348.

Bicego, T. G., and J. T. Boerma. 1993. Maternal education and child survival: A comparative study of survey data from 17 countries. *Social Science and Medicine* 36: 1207–1227.

Blau, D. M., D. K. Guilkey, and B. M. Popkin. 1996. Infant health and the labour supply of mothers. *Journal of Human Resources* 31 (1): 90–139.

Boateng, E. Oti, K. Ewusi, R. Kanbur, and A. McKay. 1992. A poverty profile for Ghana, 1987–88. *Journal of African Economies* 1 (1): 25–58.

Bortei-Doku Aryeetey, E., and E. Aryeetey. 1996. An urban perspective on poverty in Ghana: A case study of Accra. Report commissioned by the Canadian International Development Agency, Accra.

Boughton, D., and T. Reardon. 1997. Will promotion of coarse grain processing turn the tide for traditional cereals in the Sahel? Recent empirical evidence from Mali. *Food Policy* 22 (4): 307–316.

Bound, J., D. Jaeger, and R. Baker. 1995. Problems with instrumental variables estimation when the correlation between the instruments and the endogenous explanatory variable is weak. *Journal of the American Statistical Association* 90 (430): 443–450.

Braun, J. von, J. McComb, B. Fred-Mensah, and R. Pandya-Lorch. 1993. *Urban food insecurity and malnutrition in developing countries: Trends, policies, and research implications.* Washington, D.C.: International Food Policy Research Institute.

Brown, L. R., and J. Kerr. 1997. Ghana: Structural adjustment's star pupil? In *The gender dimensions of economic reforms in Ghana, Mali and Zambia,* ed. L. Brown and J. Kerr. Ottawa, Ontario, Canada: North-South Institute.

Brown , L. R., and J. Kerr, eds. 1997. *The gender dimensions of economic reform in Ghana, Mali, and Zambia.* Ottawa, Ontario, Canada: North–South Institute.

Bruce, J., and C. B. Lloyd. 1997. Finding the ties that bind: Beyond headship and household. In *Intrahousehold resource allocation in developing countries:*

Models, methods, and policy, ed. L. Haddad, J. Hoddinott, and H. Alderman. Baltimore, Maryland, U.S.A.: Johns Hopkins University Press for the International Food Policy Research Institute.

Brydon, L., and K. Legge. 1996. *Adjusting society: The World Bank, the IMF, and Ghana.* London: Taurus Academic Studies.

Burch, T. K., et al. 1987. Measures of household composition and headship based on aggregate routine census data. In *Family demography: Methods and their application,* ed. J. Bongaarts, T. K. Burch, and K. W. Wachter. Oxford: Clarendon Press.

Caldwell, J. C., and P. McDonald. 1982. Influence of maternal education on infant and child mortality: Levels and causes. *Health Policy and Education* 2: 251–267.

Cebu Study Team. 1992. A child health production function estimated from longitudinal data. *Journal of Development Economics* 38 (2): 323–351.

CENCOSAD (Centre for Community Studies, Action, and Development). 1994. *Urban market gardens in Accra.* Accra.

Chambers, R. 1989. Sustainable rural livelihoods: A key strategy for people, environment and development. In *The greening of aid,* ed. C. Conroy and M. Litvinoff. London: Earthscan.

Chambers, R., and G. Conway. 1992. *Sustainable rural livelihoods: Practical concepts for the 21st century.* Institute of Development Studies Discussion Paper 296. Brighton, U.K.: Institute of Development Studies, University of Sussex.

Chaudhri, R., and C. Timmer. 1986. *The impact of changing affluence on diet and demand patterns for agricultural commodities.* World Bank Staff Working Paper 785. Washington, D.C.: World Bank.

Christiansen, G. 1993. Sensitive information: Collecting data on livestock and informal credit. In *Fieldwork in developing countries,* ed. S. Devereux and J. Hoddinott. Boulder, Colo., U.S.A.: Lynne Rienner Publishers.

Chung, K., L. Haddad, J. Ramakrishna, and F. Riely. 1997. *Identifying the food insecure. The application of mixed-method approaches in India.* Washington, D.C.: International Food Policy Research Institute.

Cohen, R., K. H. Brown, J. Canahuati, L. L. Rivera, and K. G. Dewey. 1995. Determinants of growth from birth to 12 months among breast-fed Honduran infants in relation to age of introduction of complementary foods. *Pediatrics* 96 (3): 504–510.

Commander, S., J. Howell, and W. Seini. 1989. Ghana. In *Structural adjustment and agriculture: Theory and practice in Africa and Latin America,* ed. S. Commander. London: Overseas Development Institute.

Cornia, G., R. Jolly, and F. Stewart. 1987. *Adjustment with a human face.* Oxford: Clarendon Press.

Coulomb, H., and A. McKay. 1995. *An assessment of trends in poverty in Ghana: 1988-92.* PSP Discussion Paper 81. Washington, D.C.: World Bank.

Cox, D., and E. Jimenez. 1990. Achieving social objectives through private transfers: A review. *The World Bank Research Observer* 5 (2): 205–218.

———. 1998. Risk sharing and private transfers: What about urban households? *Economic Development and Cultural Change* 46 (3): 621–637.

Davies, S. 1996. *Adaptable livelihoods.* New York: St. Martins Press.

Deaton, A. 1997. *The analysis of household surveys: A microeconometric approach to development policy.* Washington, D.C.: World Bank.

de Haan, A. 1997. Urban poverty and its alleviation: Introduction. *IDS Bulletin* 28 (2): 1–8.

de Waal, A. 1989. *Famine that kills: Darfur, Sudan, 1984-1985.* Oxford: Clarendon Press.

Delgado, C., and T. Reardon. 1987. Policy issues raised by changing food patterns in the Sahel. In *Cereal policies in Sahel countries: Acts of the Mindelo Conference,* ed. CILSS/Club du Sahel. Paris: CILSS/Club du Sahel/OECD.

Demery, L., and L. Squire. 1996. Macroeconomic adjustment and poverty in Africa: An emerging picture. *World Bank Research Observer* 11 (1): 39–59.

Drakakis-Smith, D. 1991. Urban food distribution in Africa and Asia. *Geographical Journal* 157 (1): 51–61.

Dugdale, A. E., and P. Payne. 1987. A model of seasonal changes in energy balance. *Ecology of Food and Nutrition* 19: 231–245.

Duncan C., K. Jones, and G. Moon. 1993. Do places matter? A multilevel analysis of regional variations in health-related behaviour in Britain. *Social Science and Medicine* 37 (6): 725–733.

Edmundson, W. C., and P. V. Sukhatme. 1990. Food and work: Poverty and hunger. *Economic Development and Cultural Change* 38 (2): 263–280.

Engle, P. 1986. The intersecting needs of working mothers and their children: 1980 to 1985. Department of Psychology and Human Development, California Polytechnic State University, San Luis Obispo, Calif., U.S.A.

———. 1989. Childcare strategies of working and nonworking women in rural and urban Guatemala. In *Women's work and child welfare in the Third World,* ed. M. Paolisso and M. Buvinic. Boulder, Colo., U.S.A.; Westview.

———. 1992. *Care and child nutrition.* Theme paper for the International Nutrition Conference. New York: United Nations Children's Fund.

Engle, P. L., P. Menon, and L. Haddad. 1996. Care and nutrition: Concepts and measurement. Food Consumption and Nutrition Division Discussion Paper 18. International Food Policy Research Institute, Washington, D.C.

———. 1997. *Care and nutrition: Concepts and measurements.* Washington, D.C.: International Food Policy Research Institute.

Engle, P., P. Menon, J. L. Garrett, and A. Slack. 1997. Urbanization and caregiving: A framework for analysis and examples from southern and eastern Africa. *Environment and Urbanization* 9 (2): 253–270.

———. FAO (Food and Agriculture Organization of the United Nations). 1996. *Street food situation in Ghana.* Accra/Rome.

———. 1997. *Street foods.* Food and Nutrition Paper 63. Report of an FAO Technical Meeting on Street Foods, Calcutta, India, November 6–9. Rome.

Fayorsey, C. 1995. Ga women's autonomy: A critique of the concepts and economy of the household and family. *African Anthropology* 2 (1): 91–130.

Frankenberger, T. 1996. Measuring household livelihood security: An approach for reducing absolute poverty. Paper presented to the Applied Anthropology Meetings, Baltimore, Md.

Freeman, D. 1991. *A city of farmers: Informal urban agriculture in the open spaces of Nairobi, Kenya.* Toronto, Canada: McGill University Press.

Ga Mashie Study Team. 1996. Ga Mashie: A participatory rapid appraisal of food security in a densely populated urban community. Noguchi Memorial Institute for Medical Research/CENCOSAD/International Food Policy Research Institute, Accra.

García, M., and P. Pinstrup-Andersen. 1987. *The pilot food price subsidy scheme in the Philippines: Its impact on income, food consumption, and nutritional status.* Research Report 61. Washington, D.C.: International Food Policy Research Institute.

Gayi, S. 1995. Adjusting to the social costs of adjustment in Ghana: Problems and prospects. *European Journal of Development Research* 7 (2): 77–100.

Gebre, S. 1993. Urban poverty and food insecurity: The case of Addis Ababa. Famine and Food Policy Discussion Paper 8. International Food Policy Research Institute, Washington, D.C.

Ghana, Government of. 1996. *The national plan of action on food and nutrition.* Accra.

Ghana, MLG (Ministry of Local Government). 1992. *Strategic plan for the Greater Accra Metropolitan Area.* Volume 1. *Context report.* Accra: Department of Town and Country Planning.

Ghana, MOH (Ministry of Health). 1989. Improving young child feeding practices in Ghana. Assessment and strategy design: A summary of activities. Accra.

GSS (Ghana Statistical Service). 1989. *Demographic and health survey 1988.* Accra: Government of Ghana.

———. 1994. *Demographic and health survey 1993.* Accra: Government of Ghana.

Gibson, R. S. 1990. *Principles of nutritional assessment.* New York and Oxford: Oxford University Press.

Goldstein H. 1995. *Multilevel statistical models,* 2d ed. London: Edward Arnold.

Habicht, J. P., and D. L. Pelletier. 1990. The importance of context in choosing nutritional indicators. *Journal of Nutrition* 120 (11): 1519–1524.

Haddad, L. 1992. The impact of women's employment status on household food security at different income levels in Ghana. *Food and Nutrition Bulletin* 14 (No. 4): 341–344.

Haddad, L., E. Kennedy, and J. Sullivan. 1994. Choice of indicators for food security and nutrition monitoring. *Food Policy* 19 (3): 329–343.

Haddad, L., M. Ruel, and J. Garrett. 1999. Are urban poverty and undernutrition growing? Some newly assembled evidence. Food Consumption and Nutrition Division Discussion Paper 63. International Food Policy Research Institute, Washington, D.C.

Haddad, L., S. Bhattarai, M. Immink, and S. Kumar. 1996. *Managing interactions between household food security and preschooler health.* Food, Agriculture, and the Environment Discussion Paper 16. Washington, D.C.: International Food Policy Research Institute.

Hammer, J. 1986. Population growth and savings in LDCs: A survey. *World Development* 14: 579–591.

Handa, S. 1996. Expenditure behavior and children's welfare: An analysis of female-headed households in Jamaica. *Journal of Development Economics* 50 (1): 165–187.

Hardoy, J., and D. Satterthwaite. 1986. The illegal and the reasonable. *Development: Seeds of Change* 14 (1): 61–64.

Harriss, J., K. P. Kannan, and G. Rodgers. 1990. *Urban labour market structure and job access in India: A study of Coimbatore.* Geneva: International Institute for Labour Studies.

Hart, K. 1973. Informal income opportunities and urban employment in Ghana. *Journal of Modern African Studies* 2 (1): 61–89.

Haughton, D., and J. Haughton. 1997. Explaining child nutrition in Vietnam. *Economic Development and Cultural Change* 45 (3): 541–556.

Housing and Urban Development Associates. 1990. Housing needs assessment study. Study prepared for Accra Planning and Development Programme. Accra. Photocopy.

Huffman, S. L. 1987. Women's activities and impacts on child nutrition. In *Food policy: Integrating supply, distribution and consumption,* ed. J. Price Gittinger, J. Leslie, and C. Hoisington. Economic Development Institute Series in Economic Development. Washington D.C.: World Bank.

ICN (International Conference on Nutrition). 1993. *Plan of action for nutrition.* Rome: Food and Agriculture Organization of the United Nations/World Health Organization.

IDECG (International Dietary Energy Consultative Group). 1994. *Energy and protein requirements.* Proceedings of a workshop held at the London School of

Hygiene and Tropical Medicine, London, ed., N. S. Scrimshaw, J. C. Waterlow, and B. S. Church. *European Journal of Clinical Nutrition* 50 (February 1996).

ILO (International Labour Organization). 1972. *Employment, income, and inequality: A strategy for increasing productive employment in Kenya.* Geneva.

———. 1990a. *Strategies for employment creation in Africa.* Geneva.

———. 1990b. *Employment crisis and prospects in Africa: Strategies and options for the future.* Addis Ababa: Jobs and Skills Programme for Africa.

ISSER (Institute of Statistical, Social and Economic Research). 1995. *The state of the Ghanaian economy, 1994.* Legon, Ghana.

———. 1996. *The state of the Ghanaian economy, 1995.* Legon, Ghana.

———. 1997. *The state of the Ghanaian economy, 1996.* Legon, Ghana.

Jonsson, U. 1995. Ethics and child nutrition. *Food and Nutrition Bulletin* 16 (4): 293–312.

Jonsson, U., and D. Toole. 1991. *Household food security and nutrition: A conceptual analysis.* New York: United Nations Children's Fund.

Kennedy, E., and B. Cogill. 1987. *Income and nutritional effects of the commercialization of agriculture in Southwestern Kenya.* Research Report 63. Washington, D.C.: International Food Policy Research Institute.

Kennedy, E., and T. Reardon. 1994. Shift to non-traditional grains in the diets of East and West Africa: Role of women's opportunity cost of time. *Food Policy* 19 (1): 45–56.

Kennedy, E., E. Payongayong, L. Haddad, T. Tshibaka, R. Agble, and R. Tetebo. 1994. Impacts of credit programs on food security and nutrition in Ghana. International Food Policy Research Institute, Washington, D.C. Photocopy.

Kilson, M. 1974. *African urban kinsmen: The Ga of Central Accra.* London: Hurst Publishers.

Kraus, J. 1988. The political economy for food in Ghana. In *Coping with Africa's food crisis,* ed. N. Chazan and T. Shaw. Boulder, Colo., U.S.A., and London: Lynne Rienner.

Kumar, S., R. Naved, and S. Bhattarai. 1997. Childcare practices associated with positive and negative nutritional outcomes for children in Bangladesh: A descriptive analysis. Food Consumption and Nutrition Division Discussion Paper 24. International Food Policy Research Institute, Washington, D.C.

Larbi, W. O. 1995. *The urban land development process and urban land policies in Ghana.* London: Royal Institute of Chartered Surveyors.

Leslie, J. 1989. Women's work and child nutrition and the Third World. In *Women's work and child welfare in the Third World,* ed. M. Paolisso and M. Buvinic. Boulder, Colo. U.S.A.: Westview.

Levin, C. E., D. G. Maxwell, M. Armar-Klemesu, M. T. Ruel, S. S. Morris, and C. Ahiadeke. 1999. Working women in an urban setting: Traders, vendors, and food security in Accra. *World Development* 27 (11): 1977–1991.

Leys, C. 1975. *Underdevelopment in Kenya.* Los Angeles, Calif.: University of California Press.

Liang, K.-Y., and S. L. Zeger. 1986. Longitudinal data analysis using generalized linear models. *Biometrika* 73 (1): 13–22.

Lipton, M. 1977. *Why poor people stay poor.* Cambridge, Mass., U.S.A.: Harvard University Press.

Lipton, M., and S. Maxwell. 1992. The new poverty agenda: An overview. IDS Discussion Paper 306. Brighton, U.K.: Institute of Development Studies, University of Sussex.

Lloyd, C. B., and A. J. Gage-Brandon. 1993. Women's role in maintaining households: Family welfare and sexual inequality in Ghana. *Population Studies* 47 (1): 115–131.

Loxley, J. 1990. Structural adjustment in Africa: Reflections on Ghana and Zambia. *Review of African Political Economy* 47: 8–27.

Lund, S., and M. Fafchamps. 1997. Risk sharing networks in rural Philippines. Stanford University, Stanford, Calif., U.S.A. Photocopy.

Mabogunje, A. 1994. Overview of research priorities in Africa. In *Urban research in the developing world,* ed. R. Stren, vol. 2: *Africa.* Toronto: Centre for Urban and Community Studies, University of Toronto.

Maxwell, D. 1995. Alternative food security strategy: A household analysis of urban agriculture in Kampala. *World Development* 23 (10): 1669–1681.

———. 1996. *Methodological supplement to the PRA reports: Ga Mashie and Ngleshie-Amanfro.* Legon, Ghana: Noguchi Memorial Institute for Medical Research.

———. 1998a. Can qualitative and quantitative methods serve complementary purposes for policy research? Evidence from Accra. Food Consumption and Nutrition Division Discussion Paper 40. International Food Policy Research Institute, Washington, D.C.

———. 1998b. The political economy of urban food security in Sub-Saharan Africa. Food Consumption and Nutrition Division Discussion Paper 41. International Food Policy Research Institute, Washington, D.C..

———. 1999. Livelihoods and vulnerability: How different is the urban case? Paper presented to the Annual Meeting of the Society for Applied Anthropology, Tucson, Arizona, April 20–24.

Maxwell D, C. Levin, and J. Csete. 1999. Does urban agriculture help prevent malnutrition? Evidence from Kampala. *Food Policy* 23 (5).: 411–424

Maxwell, D., M. Armar-Klemesu, L. Brakohiapa, and J. Annorbah-Sarpei. 1997. Participatory concept mapping to understand perceptions of urban malnutrition. *PLA Notes* 30 (October): 11–16.

Maxwell, D., W. O. Larbi, S. Zakariah, G. M. Lamptey, and M. Armar-Klemesu. 1998. *Farming in the shadow of the city: Changes in land rights and livelihoods in peri-urban Accra.* Cities Feeding People Programme Paper 23. Ottawa, Canada: International Development Research Centre.

Maxwell, D., C. Ahiadeke, C. Levin, M. Armar-Klemesu, S. Zakariah, and G. M. Lamptey. 1999. Alternative food security indicators: Revisiting the frequency and severity of 'coping strategies'. *Food Policy* 24 (4): 411–424.

Maxwell, S. 1996. Food security: A postmodern perspective. *Food Policy* 21 (2): 155–170.

Maxwell, S., and T. R. Frankenberger. 1992. *Household food security: Concepts, indicators, measurements: A technical review.* New York and Rome: United Nations Childrens Fund and International Fund for Agricultural Development.

Mensah, P., M. Armar-Klemesu, D. Yeboah-Many, A. Ablordey, K. Rikimaru, K. Taniguchi, F. Nkrumah, and H. Kamiya. 1995. Microbial quality of infant foods from peri-urban Ghana. *African Journal of Health Sciences* 2 (2): 277–280.

Mingione, E. 1991. *Fragmented societies.* Oxford: Basil Blackwell.

Morris, S. S., S. N. Cousens, B. R. Kirkwood, P. Arthur, and D. A. Ross. 1996. Is diarrhea prevalence a better predictor of subsequent mortality and weight gain than diarrhea incidence? *American Journal of Epidemiology* 144 (6): 582–588.

Morris, S. S., C. E. Levin, M. Armar-Klemesu, D. Maxwell, and M. T. Ruel. 1999. Does geographic targeting of nutrition intervention make sense in cities? Evidence from Abidjan and Accra. *World Development* 21 (11): 2011–2019.

Moser, C. 1995. Urban social policy and poverty reduction. *Environment and Urbanization* (7) 1: 159–171.

———. 1996. *Confronting crisis. A comparative study of household responses to poverty and vulnerability in four poor urban communities.* Environmentally Sustainable Development Studies and Monographs Series 8. Washington, D.C.: World Bank.

Mosley, W. H., and L. C. Chen. 1984. An analytical framework for the study of child survival in developing countries. In *Child survival: Strategies for research,* ed. W. H. Mosley and L. C. Chen. *Population and Development Review* 10 (Supplement): 25–45.

Mougeot, L. 1994. African city farming from a world perspective. *In Cities feeding people: An examination of urban agriculture in East Africa,* ed. A. Egziabher. Ottawa: IDRC Books.

Multicountry Program 14 Team. 1997. Urban challenges to food and nutrition security. Research proposal and issues. Food Consumption and Nutrition Division, International Food Policy Research Institute, Washington, D.C. Photocopy.

Mwangi, A. 1995. *The role of urban agriculture for food security in low-income areas in Nairobi.* Leiden: African Studies Centre.

Nago, M. C., J. D. Hounhouigan, F. de Koning, and R. Gross. 1996. *La situation alimentaire et nutritionnelle dans les zones urbaines en Afrique.* Actes du Seminaire-Atelier tenu a Cotonou (Bénin) du 14 au 18 juin 1993. Cotonou, Bénin: Centre National de Production de Manuels Scolaires.

Naylor, R., and W. Falcon. 1995. Is the locus of poverty changing? *Food Policy* 20 (6): 501–518.

Ngleshie-Amanfro Study Team. 1996. Ngleshie Amanfro: A participatory rapid appraisal of food security in a peri-urban community. Noguchi Memorial Institute for Medical Research/International Food Policy Research Institute, Accra.

Norton, A., E. Bortei-Doku Aryeetey, D. Korboe, and D. K. T. Dogbe. 1995. *Poverty assessment in Ghana using qualitative and participatory research methods.* World Bank Poverty and Social Policy Department. Discussion Paper Series 83. Washington, D.C.: World Bank

O'Connor, A. 1983. *The African city.* London: Hutchinson.

OECD (Organisation for Economic Co-operation and Development). 1995. *West African long-term perspectives study.* Paris: OECD/Club du Sahel.

Onibokun, A. 1994. Urban research in Anglophone West Africa: Towards an agenda for the 1990s. In *Urban research in the developing world,* ed. R. Stren, vol. 2: *Africa.* Toronto, Canada: Centre for Urban and Community Studies, University of Toronto.

Payne, P. 1990. Themes in food security: Measuring malnutrition. *IDS Bulletin* 21 (3): 14–30.

Portes, A., M. Castells, and L. A. Benton. 1989. *The informal economy.* Baltimore, Md., U.S.A.: Johns Hopkins University Press.

Randolph, T. 1997. Rice demand in the Sahel. In *Irrigated rice in the Sahel: Prospects for sustainable development,* ed. Miezan et al. Bouarke, Côte d' Ivoire: West African Rice Development Association.

Robertson, C. 1984. *Sharing the same bowl: A socioeconomic history of women and class in Accra, Ghana.* Bloomington, Ind., U.S.A.: University of Indiana Press.

Rogerson, C. M. 1993. Urban agriculture in South Africa: Scope, issues, and potential. *Geojournal* 30 (1).

Rozelle, S. 1991. *Rural household data collection in developing countries: Designing instruments and methods for collecting farm production data.* Working Paper in Agricultural Economics 91-117. Ithaca, N.Y., U.S.A.: Cornell University.

Ruel, M. T., C. E. Levin, M. Armar-Klemesu, D. Maxwell, and S. S. Morris. 1999. Good care practices can mitigate the negative effects of poverty and low maternal schooling on children's nutritional status: Evidence from Accra. *World Development* 27 (11): 1993–2009

Ruel, M. T., J. L. Garrett, P. Engle, L. Haddad, D. Maxwell, P. Menon, S. Morris, and A. Oshaug. 1998. Urban challenges to nutrition security: A review of food security, health and care in the cities. Food Consumption and Nutrition Division Discussion Paper 51. International Food Policy Research Institute, Washington, D.C.

Sahn, D. 1994. The contribution of income to improved nutrition in Côte d'Ivoire. *Journal of African Economies* 3 (1).

Sahn, D., and H. Alderman. 1997. On the determinants of nutrition in Mozambique: The importance of age-specific effects. *World Development* 25 (4): 577–588.

Sahn, D., P. Dorosh, and S. Younger. 1996. Exchange rates, fiscal and agricultural policies in Africa: Does adjustment hurt the poor? *World Development* 24 (4): 719–747.

Sarris, A. 1993. Household welfare during crisis and adjustment in Ghana. *Journal of African Economies* 2 (2): 194–233.

Satterthwaite, D. 1995. The underestimation and misrepresentation of urban poverty. *Environment and Urbanization* (7) 1: 3–10.

Sawio, C. 1993. Feeding the urban masses? Towards an understanding of the dynamics of urban agriculture in Dar es Salaam, Tanzania. Ph.D. dissertation. Clark University, Worchester, Mass., U.S.A.

Sawyerr, A., and E. Bortei-Doku Aryeetey. 1997. *Ghana national human development report.* Accra: United Nations Development Program.

Sen, A. K. 1981. *Poverty and famines: An essay on entitlements and deprivation.* Oxford: Clarendon Press.

Smit, J., J. Nasr, and A. Ratta. 1996. *Urban agriculture: A neglected resource for food, jobs and sustainable cities.* New York: United Nations Development Program.

Sommerfelt, A. E., and M. K. Stewart. 1994. *Children's nutritional status.* Demographic and Health Surveys Comparative Studies 12. Calverton, Md., U.S.A.: Macro International Inc.

Songsore, J., and G. McGranahan. 1993. Environment, wealth, and health: Towards an analysis of intra-urban differentials within the Greater Accra Metropolitan Area, Ghana. *Environment and Urbanization* 5: 10–34.

———. 1996. *Women and household environmental care in the Greater Accra Metropolitan Area, Ghana.* Urban Environment Series, Report No. 2. Stockholm: Stockholm Environment Institute.

Stratton, R. J., R. J. Stubbs, D. Hughes, N. King, J. E. Blundell, and M. Elia. 1998. Comparison of the traditional paper visual analog scale questionnaire with an

Apple Newton electronic appetite rating system (EARS) in free living subjects feeding *ad libitum*. *European Journal of Clinical Nutrition* 52 (10): 737–741.

Strauss, J., and D. Thomas. 1995. Human resources: Empirical modeling of household and family decisions. In *Handbook of development economics,* vol. 3, ed. J. Behrman and T. N. Srinivasan,. Amsterdam: Elsevier.

Stren, R., R. White, and J. Whitney. 1992. *Sustainable cities: Urbanization and the environment in international perspective.* Boulder, Colo., U.S.A.: Westview.

Subramanian, S., and A. Deaton. 1996. The demand for food and calories. *Journal of Political Economy* 104 (1): 133–162.

Swift, J. 1989. Why are rural people vulnerable to famine? *IDS Bulletin* 20 (2): 8–15.

Tabatabai, H. 1988. Agricultural decline and access to food in Ghana. *International Labour Review* 127 (6): 703–734.

———. 1993. *Poverty and food consumption in urban Zaire.* Cornell Food and Nutrition Policy Program Working Paper 46. Ithaca, N.Y., U.S.A.: Cornell Food and Nutrition Policy Program.

Tienda, M., and S. O. Salazar. 1980. *Female-headed households and extended family formations in rural and urban Peru.* Madison, Wis., U.S.A.: Center for Demography and Ecology, University of Wisconsin.

Tinker, I. 1997. *Street foods: Urban food and employment in developing countries.* Oxford: Oxford University Press.

Todaro. M. 1977. *Economic development in the Third World.* New York: Longmans Press.

UN ACC/SCN (United Nations Administrative Committee on Coordination—Subcommittee on Nutrition). 1992. *Second report on the world nutrition situation.* vol. 1, *Global and regional results.* Geneva.

UNCHS (United Nations Center for Human Settlement). 1996. *An urbanizing world: Global report on human settlements, 1996.* Oxford: Oxford University Press.

UNICEF (United Nations Childrens Fund). 1990. *Strategy for improved nutrition of children and women in developing countries.* UNICEF Policy Review Paper. New York.

United Nations. 1995. *World urbanization prospects. 1994.* New York.

Victora, C. G. 1992. The association between wasting and stunting: An international perspective. *Journal of Nutrition* 122 (5): 1105–1110.

Watts, M., and H. Bohle. 1993. Hunger, famine, and the space of vulnerability. *GeoJournal* 30 (2): 117–125.

Wester, A., and T. K. Burch. 1983. Fertility and household status of older women in Canada, 1971. *Canadian Studies in Population* 10 (1): 1–13.

WHO (World Health Organization). 1979. *Measurement of nutritional impact. A guideline for the measurement of nutritional impact of supplementary feeding programmes aimed at vulnerable groups.* FAP/79.1. Geneva.

———. 1995. *Physical status: The use and interpretation of anthropometry.* Report of a WHO Expert Committee. WHO Technical Report Series 854. Geneva.

———. 1997. Prevention and management of the global epidemic of obesity. Report of the WHO Consultation on Obesity. Geneva, 3-5 June 1997. Photocopy.

———. 1998. *Complementary feeding of young children in developing countries: A review of current scientific knowledge.* WHO/NUT/98. Geneva.

Williams, C. D. 1933. A nutritional disease of childhood associated with a maize diet. *Archive of Diseases in Childhood* 8: 423–433.

World Bank. 1981. *Accelerated development in Sub-Saharan Africa.* Washington, D.C.

———. 1986. *Poverty and hunger: Issues and options for food security in developing countries.* Washington, D.C.

———. 1995. *Ghana: Poverty past, present and future.* Report 14504-GH. Washington, D.C.

———. 1997. *World development report 1997.* Washington, D.C.

Daniel Maxwell, formerly of IFPRI, is the regional food security advisor for East Africa for CARE International. Carol Levin, Marie Ruel, and Saul Morris are research fellows in the Food Consumption and Nutrition Division at IFPRI. Margaret Armar-Klemesu is a research fellow in the Nutrition Unit of the Noguchi Memorial Institute for Medical Research at the University of Ghana. Clement Ahiadeke is a demographer at the Institute of Statistical, Social, and Economic Research at the University of Ghana.

Made in the USA
Las Vegas, NV
13 April 2026

45277981R00105